C000056523

Christopher Robbins is a third-generation herbalist. Born in Australia, he qualified as a Medical Herbalist in Britain and is a full member of the National Institute of Medical Herbalists. He also has qualifications in plant sciences and has worked in the health field since 1976 as an academic, a nutritionist, the director of Britain's Coronary Prevention Group, and as a broadcaster. He divides his time between his herbal practices in Herefordshire, writing and teaching.

Also by Christopher Robbins

INTRODUCTORY GUIDE TO HERBALISM
NATURAL PHARMACY
EATING FOR HEALTH
HEALTHY CATERING MANUAL
POISONED HARVEST

THE HOUSEHOLD HERBAL

A complete practical guide to plants that heal

Christopher Robbins

BANTAM BOOKS

London • New York • Toronto • Sydney • Auckland

*For Katrina Whone, unsoppable Cerberus to the grammatical recidivist
and yet still a dear friend.*

THE HOUSEHOLD HERBAL
A BANTAM BOOK: 0553 40800 3

Originally published in Great Britain by Bantam Press,
a division of Transworld Publishers Ltd

PRINTING HISTORY
Bantam Press edition published 1996
Bantam edition published 1997

Set in 11/13pt Bembo by
Falcon Oast Graphic Art, Wallington, Surrey, Great Britain.

Bantam Books are published by Transworld Publishers Ltd,
61–63 Uxbridge Road, London W5 5SA,
in Australia by Transworld Publishers (Australia) Pty Ltd,
15–25 Helles Avenue, Moorebank, NSW 2170
and in New Zealand by Transworld Publishers (NZ) Ltd,
3 William Pickering Drive, Albany, Auckland.

Reproduced, printed and bound in Great Britain by
Cox & Wyman Ltd, Reading, Berks.

ACKNOWLEDGEMENTS

The author acknowledges:

All herbalists owe a debt to earlier generations who collected, tested and passed on folkloric wisdoms. My many patients, students, and colleagues have also left their mark on my herbal knowledge and its application. More or less of the manuscript was read critically by Amanda Eckley, Jean Saunders, Carol Cowlishaw, Geoff Lancashire and Katrina Whone. Madge Hooper of the Stoke Lacey herb garden provided stimulation and her excellent library of ancient herbals. My friend Rose Hunt created the extraordinary plant illustrations that add life and character to the book. Live and other forms of herbs were kindly supplied by Phyto Products, Hambledom Herbs, and the Herbal Apothecary. Red Cross parcels that kept me in 'treats' came regularly from Norah Parker, who also read early drafts and provided both seasonal herbs from her garden and maternal advice. My agent, Frances Kelly, risks becoming seriously indispensable for her support before and during the writing. Kate Melhuish, Debbie Beckerman, Julia Lloyd, and Francesca Liversidge of the publishers, Transworld, stroked the book through all its production stages with an uncommon and welcome calm.

The illustrator acknowledges:

The feat of portraying so many plants, most from live material, leaves me with an enormous number of people to whom I am grateful. First, and above all, Christopher Robbins, who made this project possible. To Sue Minter, Curator, Fiona Crumley, Head Gardener, all other gardeners at the Chelsea Physic Garden for patiently introducing me to their well-tended collection. To Ruth Hall who gave valuable comments and support on artistic detail. To Ginny Fraser for her generosity and belief in the project. To Chris Hedley, medical herbalist, and Malcolm Beasley of the National History Museum for help in locating the more obscure species. To Simon Stern at the Association of Illustrators, to my family and friends for their constant interest and encouragement. To all the staff at Transworld, especially Julia Lloyd whose encouragement maintained momentum.

I dedicate my illustrations to the memory of my aunt, Jessie Welch, whose love of and flair for plants inspired me from an early age.

DISCLAIMER

Herbal medicines should be treated with the same care and precautions as all other forms of medicine. Any illness should be taken seriously and self-medication used only with the confidence that comes from suitable professional advice. While herbal medicines are safe and effective when used appropriately, neither the author nor the publisher can accept liability for any consequences arising from the injudicious use of any advice or information contained herein.

CONTENTS

INTRODUCTION

To know is one thing, merely to believe one knows is another. To know is science, but merely to believe one knows is ignorance.

HIPPOCRATES.

Herbs and homes go together like knives and forks or dustpans and brushes. So much of what happens every day in every household uses either plant materials or modern industrial equivalents. This has always been so. We depend on the plant world for the simplest most essential daily functions. It is only in the last sixty odd years that modern machine production in industrial societies has seduced us into forgetting our reliance on plants, even into thinking that industrial substitutes must be better. Now we are wiser and are rediscovering the value, indeed often the superiority, of nature's plant resources in our daily lives.

Our food is plants. Try imagining even one day's meals without plant food. How about hamburger without the bun or herbs; roast meat without the vegetables; butter without the toast; not to mention no fruit, salads, herbs or spices? Medicine is the second most important use of plants. Apart from the herbal medicines that are bought or harvested for daily use, nearly half of all pharmaceutical drugs are either straight extracts from plants or are synthetic copies of plant ingredients. And many common foods, as well as herbs and spices, that are eaten daily have valuable medicinal functions.

But the complete list of the valuable uses of plants is far greater. Cosmetics, especially with the fashion for natural products, contain plants and increasingly have herb names. Aloe vera gels, jojoba oil, chamomile extract, and cucumber slices all feature in beauty products and treatments. Bath bubbles of chestnut extract are a market leader but oils of rose, lavender and rosemary are also often delightfully dripped to convert bathtime from ablution to abreaction. Plant dyes colour fashionable knitwear. Toothpaste is flavoured with peppermint or spearmint. Insecticides that protect pets and petunias contain pyrethrums or derris which come from plants. The daily newspaper and this book are made from plants. Wallpaper is made from plants as is the glue that keeps it in place. Cotton clothing and curtains should not be forgotten and nor should the house plants that decorate inside or out, not to mention the wood or coal that glows in the hearth.

With the exception of herbal medicines, these daily uses of plants are enjoyed with hardly a thought. The role of herbs in health now attracts more attention from doctors and the general public. The impetus is the increasing popularity of complementary medicine generally. An interesting aspect is that the use of herbal medicines at home is once again being seen as normal and not quirky.

Aspirin, Savlon, antacids, calamine lotion, a bottle of expectorant syrup, athlete's foot powder, and a box of bandage strips. What household, however small or grand, doesn't have most of these medicines in some cupboard or box? Doctors and hospitals have their place but self-treatment at home deals with most common illnesses. Colds, scalds, headaches, coughs and indigestion are far more common than more serious problems like stomach ulcers, heart attacks, or diabetes, which need professional treatment.

Among popular over-the-counter (OTC) medicines used at home are many with herbal contents. Vicks Vapo-rub, Throaties, Rheumasol and other rubbing ointments for sprains and aches; many cough and catarrh medicines like Olbas products and Benylin, Hypercal, and Listerine all contain herbal ingredients. There are also many OTC products that are pure herbal products, like Kalms and Quiet Life; arnica and calendula creams; Evening Primrose oil; garlic perles; and laxatives Senlax and Dual Lax.

The home medicine box is not only as common as cornflakes or kitchen tables, it is a household tradition that is centuries old. Fifty or more years ago, there were few OTC medicines. The pharmaceutical industry developed only in the late nineteenth century. Many people remember their mothers or grandmothers making herbal medicines and dosing the family. Memories are of mustard foot baths, cabbage leaf wrapped around the neck for sore throats, and elder flower tea for fevers and flu.

Plants were gathered in hedgerows, fields, and parks and taken home to dry for storage until needed, or to make into medicines. Rubs and syrups were common preparations and ointments were made from lard or dripping. Health care for most people was almost exclusively home treatment. Only one hundred years ago doctors were scarce and they cost money many people couldn't afford. Only three hundred years ago doctors were the exclusive preserve of the rich and home treatment was the only health care for the majority.

The tradition of home treatment is found in all cultures throughout the world. Whether in industrial countries or in the Third World, herbs appear in the home use of medicines, often with the same plants being used in the same way for similar illnesses.

In earlier centuries most of the population was illiterate so information about herbal medicines was transmitted by word of mouth.

There were books of local knowledge like Markham's *The English House-wife*, which first appeared in 1615. Later there were many similar booklets specifically on herbal medicine and they popped up in almost every country. Of course there were also famous herbals like Gerard's and Culpepper's. However, they rarely included the most parochial 'receipts', which often relied on local plants or traditions, and could not be read by most of the population who never saw any books and couldn't read them even if they did. A sad consequence is that much of this folkloric information has been lost as the elders of traditional communities died with their ancestral treasures unrecorded. However, there is renewed interest worldwide in herbal medicines and in home treatment.

The rebirth of natural medicine is exciting. It is not limited to a renewed interest in the professional herbalist or other complementary therapists. It appears to be based on a deep questioning of the relationships between doctors and patients and of the meaning of health and illness. The former involves patients wanting more information about their health and medical treatments in order to increase their control over their own health and how it is treated. The latter is seen as a general interest in promoting health rather than waiting for illness to appear then expecting medical treatment. Most of the natural therapies heal by encouraging the body's own healing forces, which means promoting health. Having more knowledge and control over individual health and promoting health inevitably take health care into every household.

Herbal medicine fits well into the new thinking. In professional practice, the aim is to promote and sustain health. The plant drugs are less aggressive and have fewer side effects than pharmaceutical drugs, and are chosen for their support for the body's systems rather than to suppress symptoms. But more important is that, unlike pharmaceutical drugs, many herbal medicines can be grown in the garden or harvested from the countryside, and can be prepared with no more skill necessary than that of making a cup of tea.

However, the resurgence of herbal medicines is not without opposition. The pharmaceutical companies have developed both useful drugs and a formidable marketing machine since their growth and expansion began in the 1950s. They vigorously promoted their expensive product to doctors and health service managers with such effect that faith in the superiority, safety and effectiveness of their products was greater than detailed scrutiny should have allowed. More recently, as experience of both drug disasters and the range of serious side effects has mounted, the orthodox doctors' approach to drugs has become more sceptical and questioning. Doctors reach for their prescription pad less eagerly and less often. More complementary thinking and practice among doctors is now evident.

Meanwhile, of course, the pharmaceutical companies have developed into some of the largest and most influential conglomerates in the industrial world. This means they have power and clout. They need to have large sales to keep up high profit levels and cover the costs of their research and marketing programmes. There is no denying the fact that the pharmaceutical companies have little time for herbal medicines. They can't make money out of them because they require little or no processing. They can't patent them because they already exist in fields, forests, and gardens around the world. But they can try to discredit them or encourage legislation making it harder for them to be sold as medicines.

The last ten years has seen more attempts to actually ban the use of medicinal herbs in Germany, Australia and North America. In the autumn of 1994, the latest round was fought in Britain. A government agency, the Medicines Control Agency, tried to change British law to require that only licensed herbal medicines could be sold. Some herbal products do have licences, mostly granted simply because the product had been sold for years in Britain. But new licences are expensive and, as herbal medicines are inexpensive, it would have been uneconomical for suppliers to license and sell most of their herbs. Absurd as it is, the result would have meant that it would be illegal to sell herbs like chamomile for eczema, comfrey for sprains, willow bark for rheumatism or gastritis, or elder flower for flu or hay fever. Had the law been changed, all these herbs could still be harvested in gardens or fields and used, they could be given freely among friends, but it would have been illegal to sell them. The real issue of course was that they compete with OTC pharmaceutical drugs that can be bought without a prescription.

Despite little warning of the proposed change, there was such a public outcry that the Minister for Health quietly relented. He apparently discovered at the last minute, just in time to save face, that under European Community law, herbal medicines are classified as 'traditional medicines', which do not have to go through the same stringent testing and licensing procedures as modern pharmaceutical drugs. These drugs are usually new chemical structures that have never existed before and are designed and chosen to have marked effects on the body. Such stringent testing is justified. The 'traditional medicines', however, are accepted as having been used for hundreds of years, which implies they must be both safe and efficient or they would have slipped into disuse. Herbal medicines should be monitored and researched, but the methods necessary for pharmaceutical drugs are not appropriate. Useful methods are available and are being adopted.

But be vigilant. This little skirmish was won but it is unlikely to be the last attempt to hide herbal medicines under a mountain of pharmaceutical drugs. Your choice, your rights, and your natural heritage are at stake here.

The folkloric or traditional knowledge and the thousands of useful herbs are our irreplaceable heritage. They belong to all of us and to future generations. They must not be allowed to be lost, destroyed, or degraded, whether through neglect or intent.

This book is a manual for herbal treatment at home. It draws together the lost skills of the last thousand years of home healing for use in the next millennium. The recommended use of herbs acknowledges ancient traditions but is based on current medical and scientific research. It is the most modern health guide based on the oldest of medicines.

Enjoy it, use it, keep it alive, and pass it on.

CHAPTER ONE

History of Herbal Medicine

PLANTS HAVE ALWAYS BEEN A SOURCE OF MEDICINES FOR HUMANS and other animals. Even the word drug comes to us from the old Dutch term, *droogen*, meaning dried roots.

The World Health Organization estimates that 80 per cent of the world's population relies totally on herbal medicines. Modern industrial countries have state-of-the-art pharmaceutical industries but even so, 40–50 per cent of their medicines are either direct extracts of plants or are synthetic copies of plant ingredients. From the heights of Tibet, across the arid grasslands of Africa, to the dense rain forests of South America, plants remain our most important and most used medicine.

In the last fifty years, scientific and technological advances have been breath-taking. It has been difficult to read a newspaper without news of further breakthroughs. Medicine has not been without its share. Biotechnology, and especially understanding of the genetic basis of disease, have taken medicine into procedures and treatments that were the exclusive realm of science fiction only ten years earlier. Yet in the excitement of such possibilities, our dependence on plant medicines is perhaps greater than before. None of this technology has slightly dented our dependence on plants.

The world's largest drug companies are focusing their future hopes on scouring unexplored tropical rain forests in search of new plant medicines. The plants for research back in comfortable laboratories are selected by studying the plant medicines used by the jungle peoples. The most advanced medical technologies ever known can develop new medicines only by learning from the most primitive societies living on earth. Such is the power of plant medicine.

To understand plant medicine requires understanding its history. Unlike all other technologies, new developments in medicine do not mean all previous knowledge is obsolete, superseded, or consigned to the bin if not the museum. Our knowledge of herbal medicine has been growing since records began. Although we may have refined understanding, learned of more efficient plant medicines or understood why ancient remedies work, herbalists have the greatest respect for the ancient wisdoms and uses of plants.

Much of what we know about the ancient uses of plant medicines comes from illustrated herbals and other written records. This is probably only a fraction of the traditional wisdom because most of the early users of herbs were illiterate. Anthropologists studying the earliest civilizations have pieced together other forms of evidence, such as seeds found in the remains of homes. There is a remarkable consistency of use of plant medicines throughout time and across continents.

The earliest records date from Neanderthal burial sites in Iraq. Bouquets of seven herbs have been found in graves dug around 60,000 years ago. The herbs – hollyhock, yarrow, groundsel, grape hyacinth, the yellow star thistle, and ephedra – are all useful medicinally. Evidence that the Australian aborigines also were using plant medicines dates back 20,000–40,000 years.

The earliest written evidence is the *Great Herbal* of the Chinese emperor, Shên Nung, which dates from between 3,000 and 2,700

BC. This lists 365 medicinal plants, many of which are still in use today. Although Shên Nung is known as the father of Chinese herbal medicine, many other Chinese herbals were produced. A striking feature is the number of detailed herbal prescriptions, which remain standards for Chinese doctors today. Together these works are the longest continuous series of herbal records available and were unknown to the West for perhaps 3,000 years or more.

The beginnings of Western herbalism can be found in the biblical lands of the Middle East. The Sumerian lands between the famous rivers, the Euphrates and Tigris, nurtured superior cultures who developed writing skills. Their preference for scratching into wet clay slabs or tablets ensured that more of their records survive. The oldest tablets date from around 2,500 BC and were found in protective spaces under the broken walls of decaying cities. Over 1,000 medicinal plants are listed, a remarkable feat in an arid part of the world. Almost modern by comparison are the Assyrian clay tablets dated around 650 BC. These were part of the personal library of King Ashurbanipal and listed 250 herbal medicines, including dates, figs and juniper berries as well as the seeds coriander and caraway. Willow, one of the most widely used herbs for inflammatory diseases, was also present.

Such are the quirks of history! Who knows what other cultures' herbal secrets are lost to us because they were either unrecorded or put onto crude paper which too easily decayed?

Much more is known about the Egyptians' life and times simply because of the enormous amount of recorded information that survived the desert sands. There are many records about their use of plant medicines. Tomb walls were adorned with information and among the personal possessions left in tombs were vast amounts of food, plant medicines and other conveniences for the journey. The Ebers papyrus is a 70-foot-long parchment from 1,500 BC that lists both individual herbs and prescriptions for specific diseases. Opium and castor oil are first mentioned here and many would wish this were the last mention.

Orthodox medicine also has close links with ancient history. The ancient Greek physician, Hippocrates, has been adopted as the father of medicine and is the origin of the Hippocratic oath that all graduating doctors, until very recently, had to swear to uphold. The Egyptian goddess, Isis, was the font of all medicinal knowledge. Her symbolic staff, which was entwined with a snake, has become the symbol of Western doctors. Most interesting is that both Hippocrates and Isis relied on herbal medicines.

The Bible lists over forty plant medicines. The most well known, biblically, are frankincense and myrrh. These were among the gifts brought to the stable on Christmas night. Today myrrh is still one of the most effective antiseptics in the herbalist's tool bag. Many listed herbs are widely used, even in local traditions: balm of Giliad, wormwood, aloes, camphor, nettles, garlic, cumin, cinnamon, mustard, hyssop and juniper.

The ancient Greeks were the focus of European traditions and ultimately influenced all of Western medicine. Many of the famous herbalists and their herbals emerged from the Greek and later Roman empires.

Medicine was closely entwined with Greek religion. One of the most famous herbalists was Aesculapius, who was said to be the son of Apollo, and whose daughter Hygeia gives our word 'hygiene'. The Hippocratic oath calls on doctors to swear their allegiance to the gods of medicine.

Mere mortal Greeks also made their mark. Around the time of Hippocrates, Theophrastes was busy writing his 200 or so books. He was a scientist and colleague of Aristotle. His main work, *Historia Plantarum* (History of Plants), became a standard medical textbook for the next 1,200 years. Dioscorides, another Greek, emigrated to Rome where he became physician to Nero. He was also an army doctor and travelled with the conquering armies and thus gained wide experience of Mediterranean plants. His most important work, *De Materia Medica,* lists 600 medicinal plants and was one of the most important European medical books for the next 1,500 years. He, like Hippocrates, recommended willow bark and also saw the antiseptic value of garlic and the contraceptive effects of juniper berries. These uses have been confirmed by recent scientific studies.

A greater impact on the medical profession was made by Galen, who lived during the second century AD. He adapted the Hippocratic notion of four 'humours' affecting health: blood, yellow bile, black bile, and phlegm. These were related to body secretions and were interpreted as measures of energy flow and hence of disease. Galen classified his herbs according to their influence on the humours. Thus he had hot and cool herbs, wet and dry herbs. He also broke away from the tradition of using only one or at best a few single ingredients in a prescription to what is now called polypharmacy. As the name suggests this includes many ingredients – as many as a hundred in one prescription. He was another prolific writer but most of his work was lost in a fire. His herbal knowledge escaped the fire as his book, *De Simplicibus*, which influenced medicine for the next 1,300 years. Sadly, it too eventually succumbed to fire when it was burnt in public by the sixteenth-century usurper Paracelsus.

With the collapse of the Roman empire, Europe slipped into the so-called Dark Ages. The Christians rose to power and scientific thought was discredited. Medical progress stood still. Many of the learned texts were savaged and burnt. One Christian orgy of destruction burnt the entire medical school of Alexandria, destroying its library of 700,000 books.

During these dark years, monks provided some continuity of medical traditions. They were among the most educated people in the community and their interest in the literary world left them the guardians of herbal knowledge. The monks could read Latin and Greek and translated ancient texts. Reliance on monastery gardens encouraged the cultivation of medicinal as well as food plants. Journeys around Europe as they visited other monasteries or places of pilgrimage were opportunities to gather knowledge. Skilled artists and calligraphers among the inmates left an extraordinary legacy of beautifully illustrated manuscripts.

During the European doldrums, the Arab empire expanded into

North Africa, spreading Arabic medicines and imbibing local traditions. The most notable Arab physician was Avicenna who, in the tenth century, wrote the *Canon Medicinae*. He was the Arabian equivalent of Hippocrates in Greece. His book, along with most other learned texts, was in Latin and so was read in the western and northern countries of Europe where it was influential.

Herbal medicine gained much from the monastic incubation during these dark years. The monks had collected texts and knowledge from the whole of Asia and Asia Minor. This treasure of knowledge was cross-fertilized by the monk translators and a flurry of new herbals, based on these ancient texts, began appearing from the eleventh century. The first British example of this was the *Leech Book of Bald*. Bald was a doctor or 'leech'. In the thirteenth century, the Welsh doctors of Myddfai began recording their uses of herbs. These doctors had developed their own uses of medicines from the sixth century onwards and had been influenced by Roman traders visiting Welsh ports, travelling from the Mediterranean via the Atlantic coast of France. Their 170–odd herbs were drawn from local fields and included cleavers, centaury, garlic, elecampane, mallow, and horehound. Their emphasis on local herbs was probably the first British home herbal.

A bombshell hit European academic circles during the early sixteenth century in the form of Paracelsus, otherwise known as Philipus Aureolus Theophrastus Bombastus von Hohenheim. This Zurich-born doctor shook the established views with his mixture of unimaginable arrogance and challenging ideas on medicine. His was the first serious questioning of the likes of Galen or Dioscorides for a whole 1,000 years or more. It was in acts like the burning of Galen's book, *De Simplicibus*, before the assembled professors at his university that his reputation for arrogance began. The standard medical work of the day was Galen's and many professors built their medical careers around it. Paracelsus felt that the earlier texts were based on untested theory and that the only way to treat patients successfully was to use tested diagnosis and medicines.

Paracelsus attacked the notion of polypharmacy and rejected the use of astrology. However, he revived the ancient notion of the doctrine of signatures and based his new approach firmly on it. The doctrine stated that God made plants with visible signs of their medicinal uses. Thus lungwort was used for lung infections because its leaves resembled the shape of human lungs; yellow dock was used for jaundice because of its yellow colour; St John's wort was given to treat flesh wounds because the yellow flowers released a red dye when rubbed between the fingers; the lesser celandine or pilewort has small haemorrhoid-shaped tubers around the base of the plant. He also encouraged the use of local herbs, saying that the plants were made to grow where they were needed. The doctrine may sound far-fetched but no-one knows which came first, the use of the plants or the signatures. It is likely that the doctrine simply gave religious explanations to the long-established healing powers of plants.

There came a rush of scientific herbals from the middle of the sixteenth century. William Turner's herbal was published in 1551 and within four to five years Gerard's famous herbal appeared. Both authors were doctors. In fact most of the herbals were written by doctors, displaying the importance of plant medicines to all healing.

Culpeper was not a doctor but an apprentice apothecary. He had studied at Cambridge University first and thus was far better educated than his peers. He read Latin and was able to translate the doctors' texts, whose secrets had been jealously guarded by never before being translated. All aspiring doctors had to learn Latin to be able to study the texts. The doctors were outraged by Culpeper's translation. For the first time medical books were being published in English for the non-university trained.

As herbals emerged in number and as the doctor's historic monopoly of heroic medicine was eroded through popular herb practice, dramatic legal changes were unfolding. Doctors were the most powerful professional class. They were well educated and usually came from well-placed families. In short they had political clout. Dr Thomas Linacre established the Royal College of Physicians and soon after encouraged King Henry VIII to let them have the monopoly for treating the sick in and around London. Of course this meant charging high fees and stopping local herb women and other therapists from offering their healing services at much cheaper rates. At the same time the physicians and surgeons were at each other's throats in fights over who could treat which illnesses. Surgeons then were a low class of doctor. In between these two were the barber surgeons, whose red and white poles signified blood and can still be seen outside barber-shops. On the fringes were the apothecaries who also treated the sick although they were supposed to be supplying the drugs after doctors diagnosed the illness.

A flurry of Acts of Parliament emerged as physicians and surgeons divided the available illnesses among themselves. The effect was to put pressure on what the herbalists could treat and thus the poor were being deprived of access to medicine. In their greed, the warring parties failed to take note of the country's most notable herbalist. This was Henry VIII himself.

King Henry VIII and his daughter Elizabeth I were keen herbalists, starting a tradition of royal interest in complementary medicine that is still alive today. He had invented several personal prescriptions that were used among the royal courts of Europe. The carving up of illnesses between physicians and surgeons angered Henry. It is hard to say whether he thought they might stop his herbal dabbling or whether he was concerned about the plight of the poor. It matters little. His reaction was swift and prescient.

In 1543 he introduced new legislation aimed at protecting the herbal healers. This became known as the Quack's Charter, a title suggestive of the squawks of elitist doctors as their monopoly was squashed with royal menace. The Act said that surgeons were more concerned 'with minding their own lucre, and doing nothing for the profit or ease of the diseased patient' and allowing the poor to 'rot and perish to death for lack of help'. He objected to their wish to make it illegal for ordinary 'divers honest persons as well as men and women, whom God hath endowed with the knowledge of the nature, kind and operation of certain herbs, roots and waters' to practise healing.

At face value, the doctors and surgeons were being totally self-seeking. They tried to stop ordinary people treating the sick as they had done for centuries. Henry's Act was uncompromising in stating that:

> . . . it shall be lawful to every person being the King's subject, hav-ing the knowledge and experience of the nature of Herbs, Roots and Waters, or of the operation of the same, by speculation or prac-tice within any part of the realm of England or within any other of the King's dominions, to practise, use and minister in and to any outward sore, uncome, wound, apostemations, outward swelling or disease, any herb or herbs, oyntments, baths, pultes and amplais-ters, according to their cunning, experience and knowledge in any of the diseases sores and maladies before-said, and all other like to the same, or drinks for the Stone and Stanguary, or Agues, with-out suit, vexation, trouble, penalty, or loss of their goods.

The Act was important in recognizing not only the value of traditional knowledge but also in stating that possessing a medical degree wasn't the only way to gain valuable knowledge about healing. Little wonder it became known by the derogatory nick-name of the Quack's Charter. Thanks to this law, it is still legal for herbalists to practise herbal medicine in Britain whereas in many other Western countries the medical profession has lobbied success-fully to have herbalists made illegal unless they are also doctors.

In the eighteenth and nineteenth centuries herbal medicine in Britain flourished as it did in North America. Samuel Thomson developed a system of herbal medicine based on stimulation through steam baths and heating herbs like chilli. This was similar to, if not based on, Native American medicine which became very popular as the new settlers learned more about it. This knowledge travelled to Europe and had significant influence on professional herbalists in Britain.

Herbalists like Dr Albert Coffin, who came from America, and John Skelton, a herbalist from Devon, made a large impact in the mid-nineteenth century in Britain. They produced books on herbal treatment for ordinary people and imported and sold American herbs and prepared herbal medicines. Throughout Britain herbalist shops flourished and the professional herbalist was on a crest of popularity.

The National Institute of Medical Herbalists, which was established in 1846 as the National Association of Medical Herbalists, changed its name in 1946. This is the oldest established body of professional herbalists in the world. It has spent its energies improving the formal education of herbalists and setting standards of practice. Since 1901 it has made four separate attempts to have Parliament accept the formal registration of herbalists. The influence of the medical profession on legislators, exactly as happened in the United States in the nineteenth century, has blocked the legal recognition of the qualified herbalists and their professionalism. The Institute has not given up.

Herbal medicine slipped in popularity by the 1930s. New antibiotics produced by the pharmaceutical industry made a great impact on the deadly infectious diseases like cholera and tuberculosis. These were the major causes of illness and death in crowded and poverty-stricken cities around the turn of the twentieth century. As if this wasn't enough, the demand for medicine in the two World Wars fuelled the growth of the modern drugs industry. It has now grown into one of the largest, and hence most influential, global industries.

A glance at any medical dictionary published as recently as the 1930s will show that at least three-quarters of all medicines were herbal. But suddenly doctors were barraged by expensive and elaborate marketing campaigns enticing their rapid shift to prescribing modern drugs. Herbs were labelled as 'old-fashioned' and 'inappropriate to the modern age' and doctors welcomed both the drug company perks and increased status that came with 'high tech' medicine.

By the 1970s, the tide was turning. Major drug disasters like the Thalidomide and Opren fiascos, and the growing patient awareness of unpleasant side effects from drugs, added to the realization that the modern drug approach was far from being a panacea. Nearly all of the major causes of death and illness were still incurable and the treatment was often a cause of further illness. Heart attacks, rheumatism, strokes and cancers, not to mention the common cold and flu, are still without a cure or successful treatment.

Modern drugs were no longer to be seen as the only medicine. They were shown to be neither effective enough nor sufficiently safe. Herbal medicine and other complementary therapies were resurrected from the medicinal dustbin. Sales of herbal medicines from health food shops, apothecaries, and chemists began to take off. Complementary practitioners flourished. More and more doctors began supporting the use of herbs and other natural therapies.

In European countries like Germany and France, doctors have always prescribed herbal medicine alongside pharmaceutical drugs where relevant. In Britain, as recently as 1986 the British Medical Association was still set against any other forms of medicine. Their report *Alternative Medicine* savaged complementary medicine. But in 1993 a cooler wisdom prevailed. Their report *Complementary medicine; new approaches to good practice* not only recognized the public support for complementary medicine like herbalism, it also said these professions should be registered and that doctors could consider referring their patients to registered practitioners. Most helpfully, the BMA also recommended that more research funds should be directed to studying these 'nonconventional therapies' and that doctors should learn more about them.

The wheel has turned. As though responding to renewed public interest in herbs, the pharmaceutical industry's hottest research activities are based in the tropical rain forests of South America. The most sophisticated scientific tools are directed towards learning more about the oldest known medicine. A real paradox. This neatly acknowledges the overwhelming contemporary importance of plants to the world's health.

Herbs are no less valuable now than when used by our Neanderthal ancestors 60,000 years ago. But they are not a panacea. They are effective and safe medicines, but should be used in conjunction with other drugs and treatments. True complementary healing is the only rational future. Both herbal and pharmaceutical medicines have their place. The skill of the therapist is to know when to use which medicine for effectiveness and safety.

CHAPTER TWO

Herbs for Life

THE VALUE OF PLANTS IN DAILY LIFE IS OFTEN FORGOTTEN through their familiarity. In centuries past they were more evident. Lavender and tansy were used as insecticides before agri-chemicals; horsetail fronds to clean pewter vessels before spirit cleaners were developed; lemon juice and orris root for skin care before the mega-sized beauty market; woodland flowers to fragrance rooms; indigo, woad, and dyer's broom to dye cloth.

Even today there are many uses of plants that are superior to the modern industrial products that have replaced them. Many of these plants also have medical properties that may have healed our ancestors and still have a place in healing today.

NUTRITION AND HERBS

Let food be your medicine and medicine your food.
HIPPOCRATES

There is little difference between using plants as foods to grow and stay healthy and using them as medicines to restore health. Food and medicines can be the same thing, at least where herbal medicines are concerned.

We eat foods but need only the nutrients. These are specific chemicals found in food and are essential for all animals to grow, function, reproduce normally, and repair damaged tissues. Without enough of these essential nutrients humans and all other animals become malnourished. They develop deficiency diseases like scurvy, rickets, or beri-beri. Growth may slow down and formation of bones, muscles and even the brain is defective. The immune system is weakened and infections are common. Reproduction may be impossible. Early death is likely. That's why they are called *essential* nutrients.

Out of the thousands of chemicals found in food plants, only about forty-five are nutrients. There is disagreement over how many nutrients are essential but, of all so far identified, only vitamin B12 is not readily available from plants. As science develops, new nutrients are discovered. There are thirteen vitamins, fifteen minerals, three fatty acids (the building blocks of fats and oils), and nine amino acids (the building blocks of proteins) that must be eaten for health. In addition, there must be water and a source of energy, which can come from starch, sugars, proteins or fats in the diet. In addition are disputed nutrients that some scientists say are essential but the evidence is not yet convincing: they include Factor 11, vitamins B15 and B17, coenzyme Q, para-amino benzoic acid (PABA), fluoride, vanadium, and cadmium.

Other items in food are important for health, notably sufficient indigestible fibre to ensure the bowel works easily so there is no constipation. Astronauts may live on tubes of concentrated nutrients but they still need indigestible matter to keep their bowels working. They must keep their behind in mind. Water accounts for 60 per cent of adult body weight: about forty-five litres. It makes up a large portion of the blood and is found inside every living cell. We can live for months or years without some of the essential nutrients, but only three to ten days without water.

Essential nutrients

VITAMINS	MINERALS
vitamin A	calcium
vitamin B1	magnesium
vitamin B2	phosphorus
niacin/tryptophan	sodium
vitamin B6	potassium
vitamin B12	chlorine
folic acid	iron
pantothenic acid	zinc
biotin	copper
vitamin C	selenium
vitamin D	molybdenum
vitamin E	chromium
vitamin K	iodine
	cobalt

FATTY ACIDS	AMINO ACIDS
linoleic	leucine
linolenic	lysine
arachidonic	isoleucine
	methionine
	phenylalanine
	threonine
	tryptophan
	valine
	histidine

PLUS

Energy, water, dietary fibre

But there are thousands of chemicals in plants. Less than 1 per cent are essential for life. Many are purely cosmetic in providing attractive colours or giving flavours that either invite or repel the eating of the plant. One group of chemicals, the alkaloids, give us many pharmaceutical and herbal drugs but are thought to serve no other function for the plant but to keep pests at bay as they are so bitter or even poisonous.

Some reasons for taking daily foods or drinks could be considered therapeutic. Coffee and tea are enjoyed for their stimulant effects and alcoholic drinks for the opposite, relaxing effects. The more we learn about the chemistry of plants the more is understood about the important non-nutritional role of many of these chemicals. While the number of nutrients is small, hundreds of other plant ingredients have measurable actions on the body. It is these actions that provide most of the medicinal value of plants.

At the simplest level, vitamin C is known to stimulate the intake of iron from food. Bioflavinoids found along with vitamin C in oranges and lemons make the vitamin C far more effective as a nutrient than taking pure vitamin C alone. Bitter substances in foods stimulate the digestive process by increasing saliva in the mouth, triggering the release of gastric juices in the stomach and of bile in the liver, all of which reduce the chances of indigestion. Many foods contain chemicals that gently stimulate muscle movement in the bowel to encourage emptying. There is even a range of action from very gentle (rhubarb) to strong (senna leaf). Plants like garlic, sage, and thyme contain antiseptics and antibiotics.

Plant ingredients have been shown to boost the immune system, to kill cancer cells, and to regulate the body's own hormone systems represented by endocrine glands (thyroid, adrenals, pituitary etc.). These ingredients include chemicals like alkaloids, bitter glycosides, phenolic compounds, saponins, tannins and essential oils. They are widely found in food and other plants.

The modern contraceptive pill was developed from hormone-like compounds found in the tuber of a yam plant that grows in South America. Liquorice and sarsaparilla extracts contain chemicals that stimulate the adrenal gland, which produces the body's own supply of steroids. Beetroot juice has been used in Europe in cancer treatment, but there is uncertainty about whether it affects the cancer directly rather than helping promote better health and hence the strength to resist the cancer's effects. Certainly laetrile from apricot kernels has been shown to be effective against some cancers. Some of the latest medical research on cancer and AIDS is exploring plant ingredients.

> *Ait a happle avore gwain to bed, An' you'll make the doctor beg his bread.*
> OLD DEVON PROVERB

The close similarity between the nutritional and medicinal function of plants makes it easier to appreciate how herbal medicines are used by herbalists. In daily eating the nutritional and therapeutic actions act to stimulate, promote, and sustain normal healthy activities of the body. This is also the aim of the herbalist in treating a patient. The symptoms of illness are really signs of an inefficiently working body. The herbalist uses the clues in the symptoms and a detailed history taken from the patient to discover the causes of these inefficiencies. The treatment is then designed to return the body to its healthy state by *stimulating* natural metabolism and functions using herbal medicines. This choice of herbs that stimulate healthy functions is an important difference between herbs and pharmaceutical drugs, which generally *suppress* the body's functioning.

In future, think of healthy eating not only as a means of consuming enough dietary fibre, minerals and vitamins but also as a source of natural medicinal substances to promote a healthier body and mind.

HERBS AND DIET

> *"What did they live on?" said Alice, who always took great interest in questions of eating and drinking.*
>
> *"They lived on treacle," said the Dormouse, after thinking a minute or two.*
>
> *"They couldn't have done that, you know," Alice gently remarked. "They'd have been ill."*
>
> *"So they were," said the Dormouse; "very ill!"*
>
> LEWIS CARROLL, *ALICE IN WONDERLAND*

Take any kitchen anywhere in the world and chances are that the food cupboards contain a good supply of medicinal herbs. Few are used with their medicinal properties foremost in mind, but, once known, the value of the food is greatly enhanced.

The herb and spice rack is a medicinal storehouse. Many were used first as medicine and became culinary items only through the practice of mixing the medicines with foods. One of the earliest forms of medicine used by the ancient Greeks was gruels; thick or thin soups of cereals and herbs.

Hot chilli associated with searing curries of India and tongue-stripping sauces of South America is a circulatory stimulant that stirs the very heart of the matter. The chilli is also an excellent treatment for stuffy heads, congested and infected lungs, and may help keep the blood flowing rather than clotting in the vessels. The heat of ginger brings a blush and flush to the cheeks and is used to heat the periphery in conditions like chilblains. It is also an excellent anti-nausea treatment in travel sickness and morning sickness. Very gently warming spices like cinnamon and angelica serve to keep the body heat on simmer. Most of the culinary seed spices are highly aromatic because of their essential oils which are released into the food and supply the comforting kitchen aromas. These oils are good digestive remedies, reducing wind, indigestion and colic. So dill, coriander, anise, fennel, cumin, cardamom and ajowan not only taste good, they help digest good food.

Powder for vapours occasioned by wind.

Beat to a fine powder one ounce each of tormentil and alexander roots, bay leaves and anise and fennel seeds. Sift them through a fine sieve, mix them well together, and take half a spoonful just before eating.

THE FAMILY RECEIPT BOOK, 1810

Another spice, asafoetida, is widely used in Asian cooking to aid digestion. This is the resin from the roots of two types of fennel plant. Its strong smell when raw is unpleasant to some noses and has led to the nickname devil's dung, although it is better known as *hing* in Asian cooking. Tiny pinches are added to the cooking of what are recognized as the windy vegetables (cauliflower and the cabbage family in general). It is no mere fancy that mint leaves are often added to pea soups in Europe or that summer savoury is added to bean stews and soups in North America. Both the mint family and savoury are also rich in digestion calming oils.

Pungent warming juniper berries are not used enough in the kitchen but are a useful antiseptic for the urinary tract. They are one of the main flavourings of gin, though this is not the best way of consuming the berries. They are in fact a wonderful flavouring for cabbage leaves and mushrooms. Celery seeds are rich in the oil, apiol, and are an excellent diuretic, actively encouraging the passing of uric acid to reduce the risk of gout and some forms of rheumatism.

Onions and garlic are blood and infection foods. Research studies have shown that daily garlic helps lower blood cholesterol, lower raised blood pressure, and reduce the chance of blood clotting in the vessels and causing thrombosis. Both onions and garlic are antibiotic and help destroy the bacteria causing food poisoning and lung infections. Garlic adds an expectorant action to the antibacterial bonus, making it one of the most popular folk remedies for colds, streptococcal throat infections, and chest infections. All the onion family are believed to be beneficial.

> *The greedy merchants, led by lucre, run*
> *To the parched Indies, and the rising sun;*
> *From thence hot pepper and rich drugs they bear,*
> *bartering for spices their Italian ware.*
>
> JOHN DRYDEN

Culinary herbs, fresh and frozen, offer a wider range of medicinal actions. Oregano and marjoram are useful digestive herbs. Rosemary is a good digestive and liver herb with gentle stimulation for the circulation. It is useful for headaches and also for bacterial and fungal infections. Thyme is a popular dried herb in bouquet garni and stuffings for meats. It is one of the commonest herbs grown in domestic herb gardens and many varieties are available. Medicinally its uses are as varied. It is rich in antibiotic and antifungal oils making it useful for both digestive and lung infections. The same oils are toxic to intestinal worms especially hookworms. But that is not all. Thyme is a good expectorant, which, when combined with its antibiotic properties and its encouragement of a gentle sweat, explains its reputation in colds, bronchitis, and flu. The extracted oils of rosemary and thyme are used in liniments and creams for rheumatic pains and sprains. These two herbs alone are almost a medicine cabinet.

Many culinary herbs are useful in infections. Sage and thyme are useful for gargling in throat infections and for both mouth ulcers and gum inflammation. The many mints are best known for their digestive and fever control effects but they are also helpful in intestinal and respiratory infections. Peppermint tea is a popular drink in Mediterranean countries, and an extract of its oil is the sole ingredient of a drug for irritable bowel syndrome where intestinal spasms are part of the problem. Mint jelly and sauce are traditional accompaniments for lamb and mutton and, perhaps for this use, mint was one of the plants taken to North America by the Pilgrim Fathers.

Cereals aren't only for bulk and fibre. Oats have a reputation as a calming restorative to the nervous system. The grains are responsible and explain why cereal-based milk drinks before bed or a daily bowl of oat porridge help cope with the pressures of modern living. Barley water has a similar history and is still given to convalescents to help their recovery. Cereals in general are important in the diet. They provide slow release energy in the form of starch, useful minerals, vitamins, and fatty acids as well as dietary fibre, especially as whole grains. Don't be deterred by the myth that cereals are fattening. It is the fat and sugar added to cereals that makes them fattening.

Seeds and nuts look like pills and can be as useful. Most beans contain useful soft fibre to keep the bowel functioning and anti-cancer compounds. Diabetics find pulses generally help control blood sugar, so less of the drug insulin is needed. The soy bean is good at lowering cholesterol, stops blood platelets clumping together to form blockages in arteries, and helps strengthen vessel walls. What's more, it is also rich in oestrogen-like compounds that can shift the balance in oestrogen-deficient women and may even reduce the impact of sudden menopause. Most nuts, especially walnut, are rich in low saturated fat oils that don't damage arteries and may undo the damage caused by too much animal food and cholesterol in the diet.

Sesame and sunflower seeds are rich in polyunsaturated oils that keep the blood flowing thinly and thus contribute to lower risks of heart disease. But the pumpkin seed snack, so normal in the Mediterranean and now creeping north into drinks-party nibblet-bowls, has real social appeal. They are another useful remedy for intestinal worms, this time the tapeworm, which is more likely to be found in adult parties than in schoolchildren. Be pleased when the greedy men devour the pumpkin seeds before the women get a chance as the seeds are rich in zinc and are used to treat the common, benign enlargement of the male's prostate gland.

The 1806 Edinburgh Dispensary directed that barley water should be prepared thus:

Take two ounces of pearl barley: and washing off the mealy matter which adheres to the barley with a little cold water, extract the colouring matter, by boiling it with about half a pint of fresh water: throw this water away; put the barley, thus purified, into five pints of boiling water; and boiling it down to half the quantity, strain off the decoction for use.

Compound decoction of Barley

This excellent drink is directed to be made as follows: Take a quart of the simple decoction of pearl barley, two ounces of sliced figs, half an ounce of sliced and bruised liquorice root, two ounces of stoned raisins, and a pint of distilled water. Boil the whole together till the liquid be reduced to a quart, then strain it for use. It can scarcely be drink too plentifully.

THE FAMILY RECEIPT BOOK, 1810

Fruits and vegetables are prodigious sources of health gifts. They are a gold-mine of essential minerals and vitamins, as well as other interesting properties. Apples, for example, provide vitamin C and valuable dietary fibre in the form of pectin. This helps bowel action while lowering raised blood cholesterol. The vitamin C stimulates the immune system, is an active antioxidant and has been shown to lower the chances of developing cancer, probably due to the plant acids, caffeic and chlorogenic acid. Apple juice is also a potent antiviral.

People who eat green leafy vegetables daily have been shown to have up to ten times less chance of contracting all types of cancer compared to people who eat none. Carotenes are thought to be the responsible ingredient.

Many studies have associated several constituents of fruits and vegetables with an increased ability to fight cancer throughout the body. These are carotene, vitamin C, indoles and chlorophyll. Green and red or orange types of fruit and vegetables are believed to be most useful. Thus all green leafy salads and vegetables, tomatoes, capsicums, carrots, and vitamin C-rich fruit (mangoes, strawberries, durian, gooseberries, blackcurrants, rambutans, West Indian cherries, guavas – not only citrus fruit) score high points for inclusion in the daily eating pattern.

The perky carrot has additional benefits. It softens the stool reducing the chances of constipation. It is used as a safe and gentle remedy for round worms, especially suitable in children who bring them home from school as regularly as homework.

Excellent worm powder

. . . . *if timely taken, the worms may be entirely destroyed, while the ingredients are all of such a nature, that no possible evil can arise from a very free use of them, even where there is only a suspicion that there are worms – Take a quarter of an ounce each of rhubarb, wormwood, senna, and burnt hartshorn, all finely mixed together. The dose for a child ten or twelve years of age, is as much of this powder as will lay on a shilling; to be taken in treacle, or any liquid, either last thing at night, or first in the morning, for three nights or mornings successively. Though this will often prove sufficient; it may safely be repeated, whenever there seems the smallest necessity.*

THE FAMILY RECEIPT BOOK, 1810

The denigrated and down-market cabbage is almost a home-treatment kit on its own. As well as being among the cancer protective foods, cabbage juice is a healer of stomach ulcers. It stimulates the immune system to beat off infections and has been used to wrap around gouty toes or arthritic joints and even used as a form of neck scarf to heal feverish sore throats and chest infections.

Cranberries have a strongly held folklore reputation as the best remedy for kidney and urinary tract infections. Many medical studies have confirmed this to the delight of cystitis sufferers and the comfort of doctors who can now recommend trying another herbal remedy without fearing sniggers from colleagues. The juice is drunk at a dose of one to two wineglasses a day. The active ingredient is still unknown but the juice is thought to work by stopping bacteria sticking to the walls of the tubes so they are flushed out before they can cause trouble. Blueberry juice complements it as it kills bacteria and viruses, especially *Escherichia coli*, which can cause diarrhoea. How convenient that the same blueberry juice also stops the diarrhoea while killing the causative bugs.

Herbs to flavour tea and coffee

bergamot orange oil	ginger
boteka leaves	jasmine
canella	mint
cardamom	sage
chicory root	star anise
figs	vanilla bean

The wide choice of daily drinks offer as many medicinal choices. Morning tea or coffee are both stimulants of the circulation and nervous system. They are also diuretic. The tannins in tea and the fluorides in both drinks help lower tooth decay. Both have an anti-cancer effect though the green teas of China are more effective than the black, fermented Asian and African teas. Green teas also have less caffeine, which makes them a better choice for the heavy drinker. Tea and coffee contain ingredients that relieve asthmatic attacks.

Medicinal virtues of strong coffee

Strong coffee, in the proportion of an ounce to half a pint, and particularly when made by infusion, is not only grateful to the palate, but wonderfully fortifies and strengthens the stomach, as well as the whole nervous system. It adds, maintains one of its warmest panegyrists, or gives, spirits to the body, on any sinking faintness, weakness or weariness, of mind or body, and that beyond whatever the best wine can effect; conveying as it were, life and strength to the whole frame. It is, doubtless very good against consumptions, vapours, hysterics, and all cold and moist diseases afflicting the head, brain, etc. It prevails, also, on being long and plentifully used, against the scurvy, dropsy, and gout, as well as all manner of rheumatic pains; absorbing all acidities in the whole body, and destroying the congelative powers by which those diseases are chiefly generated; while, by its diuretic property, it carries off all those heterogene and morbific humours, after a very singular manner.

THE FAMILY RECEIPT BOOK, 1810

The now popular herb teas that are drunk in great quantity by young and old, were originally herbal medicines and their benefits are to be had along with the pleasure of drinking them. Chamomile, fennel and mint teas are excellent for the digestion. Chamomile is also slightly calming and anti-inflammatory, which is why it is useful for people with stomach ulcers. Lime flower tea tastes like honey, which entices children who become calmer and more relaxed as a result. In France it is the most consumed 'tisane' and is especially valued for the overexcited child. The same merits make it the choice of bedtime drink for adults fearing insomnia. The calming effect is complemented by a dilation of the peripheral blood vessels, which is very useful in many types of raised blood pressure. Elder flower tea, one of the most popular folk remedies in Europe, controls the mild fevers of colds and flu, and is an excellent remedy for drying excess catarrh. Taken four to six weeks before the hay fever season, its strengthening effect on the thin membranes of the eyes and nose can stop hay fever attacks because the pollen grains are unable to penetrate the tougher membrane.

Elder spirit

Fill a large jar with elder blossoms, pressing them down, the stalks of course having been removed previously. Pour on them 2 quarts of boiling water and when slightly cooled, add 1 ½ ozs of rectified spirits. Cover with a folded cloth, and stand the jar in a warm place for some hours. Then allow it to get quite cold and strain through muslin. Put into bottles and cork securely.

MRS GRIEVES HERBAL

Fruit juices should be pure. Avoid anything called a fruit 'drink' as these are normally not only diluted with water but contain colourings, flavouring or artificial sweetening. Apple juice clears catarrh in the throat when drunk in the mornings and is antiviral on contact. Cranberry and blueberry juice are anti-infective in the urinary and digestive systems. Orange is usually quoted as a source of vitamin C but is not rich enough to justify its preference above other sources, especially given that many people are intolerant of oranges. The recommended daily amount of vitamin C for an adult is only 40-60mg. This can be found in any of the following: two oranges, two peaches, two apples, a quarter of a cantaloupe melon, a serving of strawberries, two kiwi fruit, a quarter of a small guava, or a dessertspoon of blackcurrants.

Vitamin C in Fruit juice (mg/100g)

apple	14
grapefruit	31
lemon	36
mango	25
orange	39
passion fruit	21
pineapple	11
pomegranate	8

McCANCE AND WIDDOWSON, *COMPOSITION OF FOODS*

Alcoholic drinks are not recommended for health but, making the best of a dubious habit, there are plenty of virtues to compensate regular tipplers. Evidence shows that the regular wine consumption in southern Europe helps explain the low death rate from heart disease there. It is thought the ingredients apart from the alcohol are responsible. Some liqueurs or aperitifs have specific medicinal properties and were probably created for that purpose originally. Absinthe was based on wormwood leaf and had excellent health credentials. It was used in nervous diseases but when abused it caused giddy fits and convulsions. Absinthe is widely banned now but wormwood, along with cardamom, angelica, fennel, and other herbs, can still be experienced as vermouth. Campari, vermouth, cynar and even the manzanilla sherry, which is flavoured with chamomile, are all bitter. This property stimulates the digestion by promoting salivation, increasing gastric secretions, and the production and release of bile in the liver. Anise in its various forms (arak, pernod, ouzo) is a calming digestive tonic.

Medieval herbals and books on household management contained many recipes for the home production of spirits flavoured with aromatic seeds, most of which combined digestive benefit with the pleasure of drinking them.

Herbs used to flavour wines or spirits

anise	hyssop
balm	juniper
calamus	lemon grass
canella bark	meadowsweet
caraway seeds	mint
chamomile	orris root
cinnamon	rosemary
cloves	sage
coriander	sloe berries
gentian	wormwood
ginger	yarrow

Bitter beers like English bitter or pilsner are flavoured with hop flowers, which convey a gentle bitterness that also stimulates the digestion. But beer drinkers beware. It has been found that beer drinkers have both increased blood pressure and the risk of cancer. Greater caution is directed to macho types who take their self image from beer advertisements: hops are an anaphrodisiac, which must be added to the disabling effects of the alcohol.

Cinnamon cordial

Cinnamon is a noble drug, endowed with many and great virtues; it corroborates the viscera, assists concoction, dispels flatulence, and is a pleasant cordial. It is, in short, cordial and stomachic; and proves of great service in alvine fluxes, and all discharges from weakness, &c. of the habit. Two gallons of spiritous cinnamon water, or cinnamon, may be thus prepared –
Take a pound of the best bruised cinnamon, two gallons and a pint of clean rectified, and a quart of pure water. Put them into the still, and digest them twenty-four hours with a gentle heat; after which, draw off two gallons with a tolerable fire. This, when thus made, is regarded as one of the noblest cordial of the shops; but, in the common way, with a pound of cinnamon to ten gallons of spirit, it is only an imposition on the buyer.

THE FAMILY RECEIPT BOOK, 1810

Of course there are many more everyday foods with medicinal virtues. Not all are sufficiently strong in their effect to justify the status of medicine. But as with healthy eating generally, it is the sum total of positive effects that make the difference between a health promoting diet, an indifferent one, and one that may be harmful as much from insufficient benefits as a long list of negative factors.

It is worth appreciating the therapeutic benefits of foods along with other good reasons why they are chosen to be part of a regular diet.

A dozen essential medicines for the pantry

apple juice	garlic
chamomile	ginger root
chilli	lime flowers
cranberry juice	parsley
dried apricots	peppermint
fennel seeds	thyme

There are many daily foods that are so effective in their healing that they are worth keeping handy for those regular minor crises like colds, scalds, headaches, skin rashes and sleepless nights. A full list of home remedies is given in Chapter 7.

WILD PLANT FOODS

Better to hunt in fields, for health unbought,
Than fee the doctor for a nauseous draught.
JOHN DRYDEN

Wild foods used to play a significant part in daily eating. Supermarkets and the burgeoning food manufacturing industry have not only replaced food gathering, they have disconnected us from the nature of food production. Young children are reported as thinking that milk comes from supermarkets and not understanding the place of cows in the scheme of things.

In the past, the relationship between wild food and medicine was so close as to be not worthy of separating. Supermarkets notwithstanding, there are plenty of easily accessible wild foods that are both enjoyable and medicinally useful. Pope's universal warning that 'a little learning is a dangerous thing' applies with strength to wild plants. Whether for use as food or medicine, please follow the cardinal rule: NEVER HARVEST AND USE ANY PLANT WHOSE IDENTIFICATION AND SAFE USE YOU ARE NOT ABSOLUTELY SURE OF. Few plants are poisonous, but enough can make you feel ill enough to warrant suitable caution. Be respectful of the need to preserve endangered plants. Remember it is illegal to remove some plants in most countries. Make sure you have the landowner's permission before harvesting.

Leaves and green tops

Green leaves or the tops of many herbaceous plants add flavour and colour to salads, and are eaten as vegetables.

Wild watercress (*Rorippa nasturtium-aquaticum*) from freshwater streams and scurvy grass (*Cochlearia officinalis*) are tangy and rich in vitamin C. The wild sorrels (Sheep's sorrel *Rumex acetosella*; Wood sorrel, *Oxalis acetosella*; Common sorrel, *Rumex acetosa*), Jack-by-the-hedge (*Sisymbrium alliaria*), and wild garlic (*Alium ursinum*) are all delicious in salads. The sorrels contain vitamin C and stimulate digestion. The garlics have similar medicinal properties to farmed garlic or onions. Jack-by-the-hedge has a mild garlic flavour but is related to the mustards. It heats and stimulates the circulation. Chickweed (*Stellaria media*) is delicate and delicious in salads with its white star flowers, and makes an efficient anti-itch, wound-healing application for the skin.

Wild raspberry (*Rubus idaeus*) and blackberry (*Rubus fructicosus*) leaves are high in tannins and are good astringents for the digestive system. They firm up loose stools. The raspberry leaves are used as a toning herb to encourage more relaxed uterine contractions in childbirth.

King of wild greens is the ubiquitous dandelion leaf (*Taraxacum officinale*). Found all over the world and a universal 'bitter' green, it can be eaten in salads or cooked as a vegetable. It is a top liver herb, perhaps the most often used herb in prescriptions by Western herbalists. The root is also used in medicine and as a caffeine-free coffee substitute. Nettle tops (*Urtica dioica*) are considered by some to be superior to spinach as a vegetable. It is a traditional blood herb that used to be taken along with goose grass (*Galium aparine*) as a spring 'tonic' to cleanse the body after the poor and stodgy diet of European winters. Of related use but different character is the gout weed or ground elder (*Ægopodium podagraria*). It was thought to have been transported around Europe by monks as a medicinal herb for gout. Now it is a weed of poorly kept gardens and waste spaces. Easy pickings for town dwellers looking for a salad herb or a vegetable tasting like celery.

Alexanders or black lovage (*Smyrnium olusatrum*) and burdock (*Arctium lappa*) offer two stem vegetables worth the trouble for the pot and benefiting health. The first was brought north by the Romans from Italy where the true lovage is native. It is a warming food. Burdock stems and roots used to appear in the popular drink, dandelion and burdock, but now has to be picked in the wild to appreciate it. The taste is not spectacular but it is esteemed as a blood cleaning herb in skin disorders like eczema and psoriasis.

Seaweeds and coastal plants

Seaweeds like dulse (*Rhodymenia palmata*), sea lettuce (*Ulva lactuca*), and bladderwrack (*Fucus vesiculosus*) have been eaten for centuries. They are tough and require plenty of boiling, but so do dried pulses so don't be put off. The most edible sea plants are carragheen or Irish moss (*Chondrus crispus*) and laver (*Porphyra umbli-*

calsi), which is eaten as a delicacy in Wales. Samphire (*Salicornia europaea*) and sea kale (*Crambe maritima*) are not botanical seaweeds, but are found growing on the sea shore. Samphire used to be picked and used as a sauce for meat where its medicinal merit as a digestive was best appreciated.

Flowers

Cowslips (*Primula veris*) and primrose (*Primula vulgaris*) have great reputations as medicines for the chest but are now relatively rare in the wild due to overpicking. They were also used to make wine. Such quantities are needed that they are best left to be appreciated in the wild. Lime flowers (*Tilia europaea*) and wild chamomile (*Matricaria chamomilla*) are relaxing herbs usually taken as infusions. The other famous drinking herb is the hop (*Humulus lupulus*) which can be found trailing up telegraph poles, fences, trees or any vertical support from July on. The flowers or strobiles look like small green pine cones and have an overpowering, resinous smell when crushed. They can also be sewn into pillows for restful sleep.

The elder flower (*Sambucus nigra*) is ostentatiously in bloom for about three weeks in May. Large, flat umbrella-shaped blooms may be twenty centimetres across. Their sweet smell is intoxicating. Famous for making wines and cordials, it has also been used to flavour cakes and biscuits. The flower is an ancient fever remedy in traditional medicine and is still a widely known and used home remedy. Many recipes for its use in medicines can be found in books.

The hawthorn flower buds (*Crateagus oxycanthus*) are known as bread and cheese in country areas where they are eaten straight from the tree. The leaves are also used as a tea. This is one of the best heart herbs available; it is used by herbalists to strengthen the heart and improve the blood supply to the heart in conditions like angina or after a heart attack.

Fruits

Country walks on warm Sunday afternoons collecting brambles for apple and bramble crumbles or pies is part of summer. Wild blackberries (*Rubus fructicosus*), raspberries (*Rubus ideas*), and wild strawberries (*Fragaria vesca*) are favourite quarry but offer little of medicinal merit. But other fruit are as easy to locate among hedgerows and are valuable. The wild dog rose (*Rosa canina*) fruit, or hips, have long been used as a colourant to confectionery and desserts. They have been used medicinally as a slight astringent and source of vitamin C. The red fruit of the may tree or hawthorn (*Crateagus monogyna*) makes passable jellies with a soft fruity flavour. Like the flower and leaves, the fruits are an excellent heart tonic. Two berries that are less accessible but extremely useful are the cranberry and blueberry. Wild cranberries are indeed native to Europe although they are usually seen only in bottles of sauce or cartons of juice imported from North America where they are cultivated. The blueberry grows on high heathland and moors throughout Britain and requires physical commitment to access its riches. Both it and the cranberry are among the best urinary antiseptic remedies freely available in nature. The elder tree (*Sambucus nigra*) is hung with large bunches of juicy, black fruits by the late summer. These are deservedly popular for home wine making. Eaten uncooked, they are carthartic and too strong for comfortable laxative use. However, once cooked, the fruits provide a gentle laxative suitable for children, adults and the elderly.

COSMETIC HERBS

Cosmetics are as old and as varied as civilization. Plants have always featured among the main ingredients and even the latest technology of the multinational cosmetic industry has not managed to dislodge plants for synthetics. With very little trouble, anyone can reap all the advantages of plant cosmetics without the high price tag or other chemicals hidden in bought products.

Cosmetics are adornments and are used to enhance the skin, hair or nails, the latter two being nothing but specialized forms of skin. Skin is amazing stuff. It is a self-reproducing protective layer that keeps the body from drying out; protects it from damage via infection, microbes or ultraviolet radiation; helps regulate body temperature; and is a sensory organ. The skin also acts as an excretory organ though only minute amounts of waste use this route compared to the bowels, bladder and lungs.

The skin is permeable to air and both water and chemicals that may be dissolved in it. Some oils can also penetrate the skin through sweat glands and hair follicles. Many medicines are applied to the skin, not only to heal the skin on contact but because they can be absorbed through the skin and reach other parts. This should be borne in mind when anything is put on the skin. The contents of all cosmetics should be safe both on contact with the skin and should any ingredients be absorbed into the body. Of course, herbal cosmetics can take advantage of the permeability of the skin by providing healing, protecting and nourishing actions on the skin.

BATH TIME

Baths are not only for cleaning. They can be peaceful and restorative slices out of hectic days. A well-planned bath should be relaxing and healing, and provides an opportunity to apply perfumes or medicatons to the whole body.

Relaxation can be enhanced by adding five to ten drops of essential oil of lavender, marjoram, geranium, sandalwood or chamomile. Stimulating or uplifting oils include rosemary, basil, juniper, bergamot. These oils are concentrated extracts from plants and should be used with care. In a bath the oils vaporize and are breathed in along with the steam, and are absorbed through the skin into the blood stream.

Herbs for baths

RELAXING	STIMULATING	HEALING
lavender	basil	calendula
chamomile	rosemary	chamomile
hops	sage	marshmallow
lime flowers	pine	comfrey
jasmine		

Dry skin is more common than oily and causes more problems. The hazards of daily living both dry and abrade skin. Ironically, many soaps and detergents used in household washing, especially baths, help dry skin. Many people have the additional annoyance of sensitive skins that can itch, sting, or flare up in rashes on contact with minute amounts of the offending chemicals. Chamomile and calendula are soothing and healing herbs for the bath. They are excellent for chapped skin, eczema, psoriasis and especially for small nappy-rashed bottoms. Mallow root and comfrey root are emollient, which means they are very soothing to damaged or roughened skin. Oat bran helps relieve itching.

Ninon de Lenclos's 'youth restoring bath'

Take a handful of dried lavender flowers, a handful of rosemary leaves, handful of dried mint, handful comfrey root, and one of thyme. Place in a muslin bag. Put bag in jug and cover with boiling water. Let sit for 15 mins then throw into bath.

Never throw herbs straight into the bath. They float and stick uncontrollably. On leaving the bath they tend to stick magnetically to you, transferring to the towel and thence to the bathroom floor. Tea bags are very convenient. Put four to six in a jug with boiling water and stand for twenty minutes before tossing the lot into the bath. The heat of the bath water alone is not sufficient to release the ingredients. Loose herbs should be infused (leaves and flowers) or decocted (bark, stems or roots) before straining and adding. Use two or three tablespoons per bath. Oat bran can be tied in a muslin bag which can be hung below the hot tap so the running bath water flows through it. The bag should be removable so it can be used as a gently medicated body scrub once wet.

Very dry skin deserves some light oils or other emollient to protect the outer layers. Cleopatra had more in mind than extravagence when she bathed in asses' milk. Cow's milk is perfect. In fact, it is far better to put the top of the milk in the bath than drink it, because of its effects on the arteries. Full-fat or low-fat milks at a good glass per bath are very soothing. Add an oil if necessary but be sparing – one or two teaspoons are sufficient. Use light plant oils like almond or grape.

Herbal soap

150g Castile soap, grated
100ml infusion of calendula and chamomile
50ml glycerine
20 drops lemon balm or lavender oil

Heat soap until melted. Add the infusion and glycerine. Allow to cool until just kneadable then add the oil and gently knead into soap. Form into tomato-sized balls and set aside to cool and harden.

Herbal soaps abound. Soap wort (*Saponaria officinalis*) easily forms a lather but is not very practical for daily bathing. Other herbal soaps are Egyptian soapwort (*Gypsophilia struthium*), Lignium vitae, and soap bark (*Quillaja saponaria*). Home soaps can be made using simple Castile soap to which glycerine and herbs can be added to suit.

Herbal hair tonic

Powdered soap tree bark	100g
vodka	400ml
bergamot tincture	20ml

Mix together and rub into hair after washing.

SKIN LOTIONS AND TONICS

Skin attention is directed at cleaning, toning and protection. In addition, it is worth remembering the perennial problem of spots and including herbal treatments among the cosmetic armoury.

Simple cleansing lotions can be based on milk or buttermilk with herbs added. Chamomile, rosewater or witch-hazel waters are excellent. Simple herbal infusions are also good on their own. If the skin is very greasy or dirty from life in cities or a dirty atmosphere at work, oatmeal facepacks laced with yarrow, chamomile or elder flowers will draw out the grime. The facepack is a form of poultice. One of mallow leaves, followed by a toning wash with apple or lemon juice, feels good and defeats the filthiest city grime.

Calendula or chamomile cream is one of the best treatments for dry, irritated faces.

Toning the skin makes it taut and helps the pores close lest they rapidly refill with more grime. The classic face adornment is artfully sliced cucumber placed on the face. Other fruits are as decorative and just as toning. Try tomatoes, orange and lemon. Astringent herbal waters can be dabbed on the skin after cleansing or used for washing. The best are sage, elder flower, ladies mantle, rose and witch-hazel.

Tired eyes are relieved by fifteen minutes under a slice of cucumber or tomato. Less restricting application of soothing gels can tone and soothe. A simple gel can be made from 100ml of an infusion of elder flowers and mallow leaves added to 25ml of witch-hazel water and 100ml of glycerine. Heat gently and add 1 teaspoon of borax. Stir well and cool before putting into jars to set. Keep in the refrigerator. Overtired or dry eyes, especially after long periods of reading, desk work or computer work, benefit from regular eyewashes with body-warm calendula infusion.

Moisturizing dry skin aims to keep it from drying out and scaling. Mashed and sieved avocado flesh is worth the effort but not recommended for wearing out of doors. Simple moisturizing creams do the job more discreetly and can be made with added medicating herbs. Most of the bought varieties have added lanolin which can cause irritations on many skins. Check the ingredients. Recipes for making home creams are plentiful but few of the easy-to-make formulas are light enough to warrant use. It can be more successful to buy a plain base from a health food shop or herbalist and add your own herbs. Most moisturisers will absorb 10–20 per cent of their weight as added herbal infusion.

Very dry skin may benefit from a heavier night cold cream. A simple mixture of beeswax and almond oil with rosewater will tackle the driest skin.

COLD CREAM	
cocoa butter	10 g
almond oil	100ml
beeswax	10g
strong chamomile infusion	25ml

Melt cocoa butter in bain-marie, add almond oil and beeswax. Add the hot infusion and stir as it cools down and starts to thicken. Pour into jars and seal.

Spotty skins usually require internal treatment to get to the bottom of the problem. But simple skin care can help. Careful cleansing and the use of astringent rinses will reduce the amount of free oil and slow down the rate of infection of the pores. Dab ti-tree oil or a strong calendula tincture on the spots to kill bacteria, heal the spot, and dry up the pore.

HAIR

Most shampoos are too brutal for hair and leave it denuded of natural oils. Conditioners are necessary to rectify the damage by coating the hair with chemicals just after you have spent time and energy washing other chemicals away. The best cosmetic is to choose the gentlest shampoo possible.

Herbs can help. Hair condition is improved by rinsing with elder flower, nettle or sage infusions. Greasy hair benefits from astringents like horsetail, yarrow and witch-hazel.

Itchy scalp may be due to dirty skin or dandruff. Allergies, infections or irritants cause inflammation of the skin, which dries and flakes. Chamomile and calendula infusions, to which a few drops of ti-tree oil have been added, ease the itch and can heal the irritation. More stubborn flaking benefits from the addition of thyme and lavender oils to the infusion, massaging it into the scalp daily for a week.

Baldness and thinning hair has many causes. Nutrient deficiencies cause general thinning but discrete patches of hair loss are often due to infection or the nervous pulling out of the hair, often without realizing it. A rinse containing rosemary, which stimulates the circulation, may be all that is needed to increase the blood flow to the hair follicles and arrest hair loss.

TEETH, GUMS AND BREATH

Plastic toothbrushes and handy tubes of toothpaste boasting countless flavours are a modern convenience. Not much beyond a hundred years ago toothbrushes were a luxury and powders or charcoal were used as 'dentifrices'. Today salt is about as good as is available for cleaning. Fluoride aside there is nothing special about modern toothpaste.

Liquorice root makes a soft and healthy toothbrush. It has the added advantage of tasting pleasant and containing anti-inflammatory ingredients that help soothe inflamed gums. Convenient anti-scorbutic brushing is offered by horseradish roots.

Tooth stain can be removed by rubbing the teeth with sage leaves or split strawberries, especially the wild variety. Do not rub the teeth with lemons as the acidity quickly erodes the protective enamel layer.

Bad breath is often mere vanity. True halitosis can be due to rotting food in tooth cavities, to infections in the teeth and throat or to digestive problems. Once the infective causes have been checked, simple fresheners of plant seeds are effective for short-term confidence, especially after eating strong foods. Try cardamom, dill, fennel, or anise seeds chewed during the day. Cloves have been used for thousands of years. Hold one in the mouth during the day. Its antiseptic properties will help destroy the bacteria causing rotting food odours.

Many herbs have been used for the dreaded toothache. A few drops of clove or oregano oil is effective but try chewing some prickly ash bark or fresh ginger root.

> *Nutmegs cause a sweet breath, and mends those that stinke, if they be chewed and holden in the mouth.*
> GERARD'S HERBAL, 1636.

Gingivitis or inflamed gums can be treated with gargles of sage, tormentil or powdered oak bark. The latter is strong enough to get rid of mouth ulcers for those who cannot handle the bitterness of tincture of myrrh, one of the best contact antiseptic herbs known. Sage gargle is also both astringent and antiseptic, helping with sore gums and throat.

ROOM FRESHENERS

Forget the synthetic chemical fresheners in plastic boxes or aerosol-driven cans. Herbs provide an enormous variety of perfumes and are attractive as well.

Traditionally herbs were strewn on the floor to kill insects or simply combat the odour of crowded living in relatively unhygienic conditions. Lavender, tansy, southernwood, wormwood, and oregano kept insects from the clothes box or wardrobe. Boxes of cedarwood, camphorwood, or sandalwood are rich in resins and oils that provide insect repelling aroma.

Where aroma was the main purpose, potpourri was used and are still popular. All plant parts have found their way into favourite recipes where mixtures of flowers, leaves, bark, seeds and extracted oil are combined. Because the potpourri is left in rooms so its vapours can diffuse continuously into the air, part of their art is their appearance. Mixtures of blended colours or mounting the whole mixture in shapes like balls tied in matching ribbons provide an acceptable display of what after all is otherwise a collection of dead leaves that would be thrown out.

There are two main types of potpourri. The moist method is the original. Here partly dried flowers and leaves are packed in layers with salt which draws out and retains the scented moisture of the herbs. After some weeks, the mixture is extended by the addition of other dried herbs or oils. The dry method is more immediate and less messy. Dried herbs are combined with fixatives, which are usually resinous plant extracts like benzoin or storax or roots like orris. The fixative helps retain the scent of the mixture and contributes its own perfume. A well-made potpourri can last two to three years.

Herbs for potpourri

FLOWERS		SEEDS AND FRUITS
carnations		juniper
elder flower		cloves
honeysuckle		nutmeg
sweet peas		vanilla
lavender		allspice
lemon-scented geranium		orange peel
rose		

LEAVES	BARKS AND WOOD	FIXATIVES
bay	cinnamon	benzoin
bergamot	pine chips	frankincense
melilot	sandalwood	myrrh
rosemary		orris root
rue		salt
sage		sweet flag root
sweet vernal grass		tonka beans
thyme		

Apart from potpourri there are other ways of bringing herb perfumes into the home. Essential oils from a wide range of plants are available. These are highly perfumed and one or two drops among the blankets, in the linen cupboard, in the final rinse of the washing machine, or vaporized in an aromatherapy burner, transform the air. Scented plants can be grown indoors or outside around the windows and doors. Honeysuckle and sweet jasmine are two favourites.

DYEING WITH HERBS

The most famous but least recognized plant dye must be indigo. Denim for the original blue jeans was dyed with indigo, which is particularly resistant to sun bleaching. Modern jeans cheat with synthetic dyes.

Dyeing is as old as civilization. The ancient methods are still the basis of modern dyeing procedures, many of which still rely on plant dyes. All cloth dyeing relies on suitable dyes and special chemicals known as mordants that bind with both the cloth and the dye-making a more permanent 'fixing' of the colour. Most mordants are salts of metals like aluminium, potassium, iron, chrome or tin. Mordants are usually applied to the cloth before adding the dye.

Plants provide a wide range of colour choice and the final colour can be manipulated by the choice of mordant and blending of dyes. Many common plants give interesting colours and can be used easily.

Plant dyes

PLANT	COLOUR	MORDANT
agrimony	yellow	alum
blackberry	tan	alum
coltsfoot	green-yellow	alum
dandelion root	magenta	alum
dyer's broom	yellow	alum
elderberries	purple	alum
golden rod	yellow	tin
ladies bedstraw	rust	alum
madder	red	alum
meadowsweet	black	alum
nettle	grey	alum
onion	ochre	copper
st john's wort	beige	alum
weld	yellow	alum
woad	blue	sodium

CALMING HERBS

Keeping calm and relaxed is not as easy as taking something to encourage relaxation. Put the heavy drugs aside, there are many varied herbal relaxants. But there is more to calming herbs than simple relaxants. The professional herbalist can select forms of action on the nervous system. Relaxing herbs calm the central nervous system as though unknotting tensions. Sedatives of varying strengths dull the sensitivity and operation of the nervous system to induce sleep or stop pain. Hypnotics are not herbs for party tricks but herbs that encourage sleep. Antispasmodics relieve tension in muscles, which is a consequence of stress and can cause pain or disturbance of normal bodily functions. There are also herbal anti-depressants, tranquillizers and stimulants. From this stress pharmacy are simple and safe calming herbs for daily use.

Although tea or coffee are drunk daily as a 'pick-me-up', they are also reached for to relax. This is odd since both drinks contain caffeine and other strong stimulants. Tea before bed or during the night is hardly the best choice for insomniacs. Lime flower, verbena, and lemon balm teas are among the best calming teas. All are safe for children. Commercial mixtures are available and usually contain one or more of the above perhaps with skullcap, hops, passion-flower leaf, and valerian root. Such mixtures are aimed at a wide range of nervous system problems.

Foods can be calming. Oats are used as a calming food and a daily bowl of porridge or oat-based museli is a good start. Lemon balm leaves can be added to salads. Lettuce, especially mature crispy leaf types containing plenty of white latex or sap is very calming. Usually the few leaves eaten in a salad do not provide enough of the sap, but try braising the whole lettuce or making lettuce soups.

Baths are a well-tried refuge of the stressed. The hot water and silence do wonders. But try adding 5-10 drops of lavender, chamomile, neroli, or sandalwood oil.

Restless stomachs usually tell their owners when they need

calming. It is amazing how quickly stress disrupts the digestion. Much of the common condition called irritable bowel syndrome is due to stress alone. As well as trying the calming teas above, take herbs to calm the stomach and digestive tract. Chamomile and mint teas, or the aromatic seeds, fennel, dill, coriander, caraway and anise, used either as teas after food or added to food are excellent. Strong cramping spasms of the large bowel purr gently in response to valerian tincture or lemon balm tea.

Tense necks and nervous spasms in the muscles of the spine respond well to gentle massage with oils containing lavender, which is antispasmodic as well as helping calm the whole nervous system.

Tension headaches can be relieved with the help of general calming herbs but wood betony has a special affinity for headaches. Some types of migraine, notably the 'hot' migraines due to constricted blood vessels, respond well to feverfew.

Sleep patterns go haywire under stress. There are few things as unhelpful to a stressed body as having broken sleep and waking exhausted and washed-out in the morning. Sleep problems can be due to anxiety, depression, exhaustion, pain, or simply being a light sleeper. Choose herbs accordingly. Anxiety responds to skullcap combined with some calming valerian. Light sleepers may need sedatives like hops or Californian poppy, perhaps combined with passion flower as a hypnotic. Exhausted sleepers are eased back into restorative sleep with verbena, oats and gentle relaxants of which lime flower, lemon balm or valerian could be chosen. For children use passion flower and lime flower, both of which are safe and gentle in their effects.

One of the best features of herbal calming is that there is no addiction and no side effects. Anyone used to drugs like valium or any of the sleeping drugs will know of the side effects and the oppressive hung-over feeling in the morning. Herbs present none of these problems.

PLANT OILS

Extracted plant oils are big business. Many seed crops provide the fixed oils which are important in foods and cooking. These oils are complex chemical mixtures of building blocks called fatty acids, the different combinations of which give the oils their specific properties. Palm and coconut oils are saturated but soya, sunflower, maize, walnut, safflower and olive are all unsaturated. Some oils are rich in particular fatty acids that make them useful for medicine as well as for food. Borage and evening primrose oils contain high concentrations of gamma linolenic acid (GLA) which has been found useful in some types of eczemas, arthritis and premenstrual syndrome.

Essential oils are volatile oils found widely in plants. They are mixtures of chemicals and supply the aroma of plants. Many essential oils are medicinally valuable. The oils in aromatic spices are the ingredients that help relax the digestive tract and soothe colic. Thyme, hyssop and sage contain highly antiseptic oils. Camphor has skin-heating oils that are useful in arthritis and sprains, while chamomile and arnica are rich in anti-inflammatory oils. In fact the medicinal actions of these essential oils make them a pharmacy all on their own.

Aromatherapy uses essential oils that are both the source of the 'aroma', as well as delivering the therapeutic action through the skin and when breathed in during the massage.

INSECTICIDE AND PESTICIDES

Two of the most widely used commercial insecticides are pyrethrum and derris. Both come from plants. This should not be surprising as plants have evolved clever methods of avoiding being eaten by insects. Walk in any garden and you will notice that some plants seem not to be attacked at all while others resist all but one or two insects. In nature, few plants are devastated by insects, so there must be something we can learn from the plant world to keep insects at bay.

The ancients used lavender, fleabane, and tansy as strewing herbs. Fresh leaves were scattered on the floors and not swept up for weeks. As they dried and footsteps repeatedly squashed them, insect repellent oils were released. Flies and cloth-eating moths were kept at bay. Until the early twentieth century, wardrobes contained ornamental porcelain or cloth containers of lavender flowers to repel insects.

Strong insecticides can be made from pyrethrum, derris, quassia wood chips, tobacco, and wormwood. Crushed garlic bulbs and chopped rhubarb leaves are insecticidal.

Flies and midges can be repelled by hanging a crushed leaf of elder over the ears or, more conveniently, splashing a strong infusion of elder leaf on the skin. Oil of lavender and citronella are powerful insect repellents for the skin.

Companion planting in the garden is a clever way of mixing repelling plants with plants that would otherwise attract certain insects. Spring onions planted among the lettuce, beans and even ornamentals indoors repel white and green fly. When mature the onions can then be eaten. Chives and garlic also repel aphids, and chives especially have a fungicide effect, protecting roses from black spot. Hyssop is a useful cough herb that can be planted among the lettuce to keep aphids away. French marigold and nasturtium chase white fly from indoor tomatoes.

Tansy and wormwood are beautiful garden plants. They repay an invitation to grow by repelling moths and flies. Cut and scattered leaves deter snails and slugs. Sage bushes on the edge of the vegetable patch will keep cabbage white moths away.

Indoors, mint leaves placed in the larder will keep mice away. Rabbits are deterred by a wall of mint around the vegetable patch but the guarantee rapidly self-destructs as rabbit food supplies dwindle.

Cat and dog fleas hate onion. Plant leeks, garlic or onions around cat paths. Brush pets with a brush that has been stroked across the cut surface of an onion. The smell soon dissipates, but not as fast as any resident fleas. Rue, tansy and wormwood also repel fleas and can be planted in the garden, scattered in animal bedding, or massaged into the coat. Southernwood, a relative of wormwood, powdered and scattered on carpets and floors will keep fleas out of the house.

Head lice can be killed with a strong infusion of quassia chips and phytolacca bark. An infusion of wormwood to which eucalyptus oil is added also kills lice and nits.

CHAPTER THREE
Traditional Formulas & Remedies

REMEDIES PASSED DOWN THROUGH FAMILIES OR FOUND IN OLD books are often dismissed as 'old wives' tales'. These three words, usually delivered thoughtlessly, are meant to have our folkloric knowledge consigned to the dustbin. In Western societies, 'old' people and 'old' ideas have little value; 'wives' have little status; and 'tales' are either fictions or lies. This is a perverse treatment for a medicinal heritage that is not only used regularly in every home but remains the core of the drugs found in the most modern pharmacy.

A dose of honey and lemon juice for a head cold or drinking chamomile tea to ease indigestion are typical of time-tested, true home remedies. Even the most widely used pharmaceutical painkiller, aspirin, is little more than a minor variation of an ancient traditional remedy.

In medicine, there is little that is genuinely new and modern. The majority of illnesses are still diagnosed on criteria that have been known for centuries. The most commonly used drugs, whether by doctors or in over-the-counter medicines we buy from chemists or health food shops, are based on old knowledge. Even modern antibiotic drugs may have been in production for twenty or thirty years. Nearly half of all modern drugs are based on plant medicines that have been in use for perhaps thousands of years.

One of the most famous examples is the origin of digoxin, the standard pharmaceutical drug for heart failure. An English doctor, William Withering, is credited with 'discovering' the value of the foxglove (*Digitalis purpurea*) in treating dropsy. This was the name for the oedema or accumulation of water, a symptom of many conditions including heart failure. In fact, he simply conducted experiments on one particular ancient, traditional remedy and wrote it up as *An account of the foxglove*. He found that an old herb woman in the English county of Shropshire had been treating dropsy successfully with a herb formula that included foxglove leaves, among more than twenty plant ingredients. Withering was particularly interested in the role of foxglove, which, he noted, had been used elsewhere as both a cure for dropsy and a diuretic among other unrelated uses.

After ten years of experimenting, Withering built up a dossier of case studies that convinced him that an extract of the leaves could be used safely as an effective treatment for dropsy. He didn't realize then that dropsy was only a symptom and not a disease. It was years later that heart failure was learned to be one of the main causes of dropsy. The foxglove drug worked on these patients by increasing the strength of the heartbeat in the failing heart.

Experienced Excellent Receipt for a Dropsy.

Taken by Lady Betty Bedingfield; and to have proved successful, after the artichoke medicine and several others compleatly failed —Boil three handfuls of the tops of green broom, in a gallon of spring water, and keep taking off the scum as long as any continues to rise; then after letting it stand till cold, pour the broom and concoction together into an earthen jug, and keep it closely covered for use. Take every night and morning, a large spoonful of unbruised mustard seed; and, immediately after swallowing it, drink half a pint of the broom water.

THE FAMILY RECEIPT BOOK, 1810

History books credit Withering with the discovery of foxglove. They play down the essential fact that he borrowed an existing medicinal formula, which included foxglove as an established traditional treatment for dropsy. The general success of the old herb woman's formula may have been due to the other herbs present as well as to the foxglove. The causes of dropsy include anaemia, liver and kidney disease, lymphatic obstruction and heart failure. Her formula may have been useful against several of the causes at once.

FORMS OF TRADITIONAL REMEDIES

Traditional remedies are found in several forms. Patent or licensed medicines can be bought in health food shops and chemists. Herbs were known as 'simples' when they were used alone. Rubbing dock leaves on nettle rash or applying a comfrey poultice to a sprain are typical examples. The old herbalists called this use of herbs 'simpling' and even they thought it an odd choice. Gerard offered his own herbal as '. . . The drift whereof is a ready introduction to that excellent art of simpling, which is neither so base nor contemptible as perhaps the English name may seem to intimate.'

The most interesting are the old formulas or receipts, where several herbs were combined, often under special instructions, to produce special medicines. Many of these formulas became patent medicines.

Fox's Marshmallow Pomade

A peculiar combination of marshmallow, petroleum, and cantharides. For encouraging and stimulating the growth of the hair, rendering it healthy, luxuriant, and glossy, and preventing its coming out or turning grey. Sold in 1/- and 6d jars.

Some may appear bizarre or just incomprehensible to us today. The food writer M.F.K. Fisher's favourite work was a collection of folk remedies, *A cordial water*. She quotes the following receipt, supposedly from a London apothecary living in Shakespeare's time:

> *For a consumption*
> *Take 30 garden snails & 30 Earth worms of middling sise, bruise*
> *ye snails & wash them & ye worms in fair waters, cut ye worms in*
> *pieces. Boil these in a quart of Spring water to a pint. Pour it boil-*
> *ing on to 2 ounses of Candied Eringo root sliced thin. When it is*
> *cold strain it thro a fine flannel bag. Take a quarter of a pint of it*
> *warm, with an Equal Quantity of Cow's milk till well, at twilight.*

Less unwelcoming but just as curious is this gem from a household herbal of the 1880s. Described as a Northern Remedy for deafness, it advises:

> *After well syringing the ears, so as to free them from the wax, fif-*
> *teen drops of laudanum are put into each; and, a cake composed of*
> *three parts rye flour and one part finely pounded juniper berries,*
> *mixed up with a sufficient quantity of vinegar, being made and*
> *baked, when the party is ready for bed, the hot cake is split in two,*
> *and applied over each ear, well covered with flannels. By this*
> *means the head is kept in a continued and free perspiration for*
> *several hours; and on removal of the cake, the hearing is commonly*
> *found fully restored.*

While we may either marvel or chuckle at such remedies, they may well be based on good empirical evidence and have a physiological explanation. Excess ear wax is a common cause of partial deafness. The syringing of the wax plus the use of the cake 'hot water bottle' to soften and help expel any remaining wax around the eardrum should indeed be effective. It would not help deafness caused by damage to the nerves within the ear, but deafness due to blocked ears was common enough.

Patent medicines were popular in the eighteenth and nineteenth centuries. Some, like Fox's Marshmallow Pomade, faded away with the Edwardian era but others remain. Coughs and colds are a common excuse for buying over-the-counter remedies today. Potter's Vegetable Cough Remover is as popular as any. This delicious mixture contains eight well-known herbs aimed at relieving most types of cough. Patent medicines are rarely original but make easily available well-tried formulae. Potters also market Life Drops. These were a patent medicine originally formulated and sold by Herefordshire herbalist, Wilf Pigott, from 1936 as Lyph Dropine. His formula (*Capsicum*, elder flower and bryony) was based on ancient practice.

Lyph Dropine

The greatest known cure for Influenza, Bronchitis, Pneumonia, Cramp, Coughs and Colds.

As a preventive, this is the surest and safest known. Being a powerful Heart Tonic and Stimulant, it is effectual in many Heart and Nerve Diseases. For Flatulence and Colic this is Nature's Medicine Par excellence.

DOSE: 2-5 drops in a cup hot water, adding sugar.

W PIGOTT, HEREFORD, 1936

Not all these ancient remedies were approved of in their time. It should not come as a surprise to discover the old herbalists mocking silly treatments. Gerard, whose herbal is one of the wittiest and most enjoyable to read, gave no time to fanciful claims. Mandrake has always been associated with magic. It was said that the roots were shaped like men, and that on uprooting the plant not only could human shrieks of pain be heard but that the person uprooting the plant would soon die. Gerard mocked these ideas as '. . . ridiculous tales brought of this plant, whether of old wives, or some runnagate Surgeons or Physicke-momgers I know not, (a title bad enough for them) but sure some one or moe of them that sought to make themselves famous and skillful above others, were the first brochers of that errour I speak of.'

Gerard explained that the claims must be folly since he and his servants had dug up and even replanted many mandrake plants without seeing any roots shaped like men and, obviously, without dying. He claimed 'idle drones that have little or nothing to do but eate and drinke' had carved the roots of bryony into the shapes of men 'to confirm the error amongst the simple and unlearned people'.

The ancient Greeks made many fanciful claims of the peony. It was said that if any man were to pick it in daylight and be seen by a woodpecker, he would surely lose his eyes to the bird. Gerard dismissed this as 'vaine and frivolous'. Larkspur's hopeful property of rendering poisonous scorpions weak and harmless, and the notion that plantain roots hung about the neck would cure grief or other diseases were dismissed as 'frivolous toyes'.

Daffy's elixir

For colicky pains take:

5oz aniseeds	3oz elecampane
3oz fennel	7oz jalap
4oz parsley seeds	21 drachms saffron
6oz spanish liquorice	6oz manna
5oz senna	2 lb raisins
1 oz rhubarb,	1/4oz cochineal
	2 galls brandy.

Stone the raisins, slice the roots, and bruise the jalap. Then mix the whole together; and after letting them stand close covered for 15 days, strain out the elixir.

TRADITIONAL REMEDY

Were these claims the product of ignorance and superstition or were they the first recorded false and misleading marketing claims? Gerard says several times that both the ancient Greeks and Egyptians were known to fake claims to increase their status. It is also possible that many were a form of product protection. By creating confusing or threatening rituals around the preparation of medicines and the art of healing, ideas and skills could not be copied easily. The same tricks with information and product claims can be seen any day among the feast of TV advertisements.

Just reflect on the supposed virtues of the different washing powders or cars on offer.

The old medieval herbalists also managed to exercise a sense of humour while transmitting their widely gathered knowledge. Culpeper was notorious for his criticisms of physicians but didn't spare his herbal colleagues when the opportunity arose. Having described at length the many virtues of cinquefoil, he concludes by noting that: 'Some one holds that one leaf (of cinquefoil) cures a quotidian, three a tertian, and four a quartian ague, and a hundred to one if it not be Dioscorides, for he is full of such whimsies.'

Also, in his herbal, Culpeper mocks those who make exaggerated claims of clary to heal 'weak backs' and the consequences, namely the 'running of the reins' (kidneys) in men or 'the whites' in women. He jests that many run to the clary bush in the garden at the first sign of kidney disease or leucorrhoea shouting: 'Maid, bring hither the frying pan, and fetch me some butter quickly. Then they will eat fried clary just as hogs eat acorns, and this they think will cure their disease forsooth! Whereas, when they have devoured as much clary as will grow upon an acre of ground, their backs are much the better as though they had never touched it – nay, perhaps, very much worse. We will grant that clary strengthens the back; but this we do deny, that the cause of the running of the reins in men, of the whites in women, lies in the back, though it sometimes be weakened by them; and therefore for medicine is as proper for me, when my toe is sore, to lay a plaster on my nose.'

Social conscience, and awareness of wife battering in particular, is sometimes seen as a twentieth-century phenomenon. Nonsense. Gerard clearly had his tongue firmly wedged in his cheek when he said of Solomon's seal that: 'The root stamped while it is fresh and greene, and applied, taketh away in one night, or two at the most, any bruise, blacke or blew spots gotten by fals or womens wilfulnesse, in stumbling upon their hasty husbands fists, or such like.'

Most of the traditional remedies have been in use for centuries. Often the same herbs, or very close relatives, have been found being used for the same conditions in different parts of the world. Many are not only still in use as traditional remedies but have found their way into pharmaceutical drugs. It is difficult to dismiss the importance of this ancient knowledge when at least 80 per cent of the world's population still rely on herbal medicines and about 40 per cent of all modern pharmaceutical drugs are either extracts of herbs or synthetic copies of plant ingredients, sometimes with minor modifications. There must be some reason to believe they are effective and safe.

Pleasant Emulsion for a Cough, Cold or Hoarseness.
Mix half a pint of hyssop water, half an ounce of oil of almonds, two ounces of powdered loaf sugar, and a teaspoonful of hartshorn. Take a table-spoon full every night and morning. If there be any rawness or sore-ness of the throat or breast, add two tea-spoonfuls of Friar's balsam or turlington's drops.

THE FAMILY RECEIPT BOOK, 1810

Syrup and Oxymel of Garlic, for Old and Asthmatic Coughs
The syrup of garlic, though one of the least pleasant syrups which is made, gives the virtues of garlic in the best manner they can possibly be acquired and retained by means of any watery menstrum. Macerate one pound of sliced garlic, in a closed vessel containing two pounds of boiling water, for twelve hours; and add four pounds of double-refined sugar to the strained liquor. This syrup may be advantageously taken, a tea-spoon or two at a time, in obstinate coughs, whenever they are troublesome; and it is particularly adapted to be used on such occasions during the night.
For the oxymel, boil a quarter of an ounce each of caraway and sweet fennel seeds, in a glazed earthen vessel containing about half a pint of vinegar; when they have boiled a short time, add an ounce and a half of garlic cut in slices, cover the whole closely up, and let it stand till cold. The liquor must then be expressed; and mixed with half a pound of clarified honey. This medicine, if persisted in, will frequently, is said, not only relieve, but absolutely cure, an old asthmatic cough.

THE FAMILY RECEIPT BOOK, 1810

> *Powder for Vapours occasioned by Wind*
> *Beat to a fine powder one ounce each of tormentil and alexander*
> *roots, bay leaves, and anise and fennel seeds. Sift them through a*
> *fine sieve, mix them well together, and take half a spoonful just*
> *before eating. This is said to have cured a person who had many*
> *years tried other medicines.*
>
> THE FAMILY RECEIPT BOOK, 1810

The very nature of traditional remedies contains an effective testing procedure – experience of trial and error. This is also known as empiricism, which means knowledge through observation and experiment. Empirical knowledge is thus what we know we know. Experience may show that a remedy works every time but we may not know why it works. There may not even be a theory of how the remedy could work.

> *That which might be written of this herbe Solomon's seal as touching the*
> *knitting of bones, and that truely, would seeme unto some incredible; but*
> *common experience teacheth, that in the world there is not to be found*
> *another herbe comparable to it for the purposes aforesaid: and therefore in*
> *brief, if it be for bruises inward, the roots must be stamped, some ale or*
> *wine put thereto, strained, and given to drinke.*
>
> GERARD'S HERBAL, 1636

However satisfying it may be to be able to explain how a remedy works, not being able to explain doesn't make it less effective. The more that is known about disease and about how herbs and other medicines work, the more likely it is that new uses of herbs or of chemical drugs can be suggested and then tested in specially designed experiments. This is the area of medical discovery. The history of medicine is about observation and empiricism.

There have always been amazing theories of the causes of disease and of how medicines worked. Most are now considered laughable, even though they were widely accepted in their day, often by the most learned members of society. Less ridiculed are the centuries of observation of traditional remedies.

The empirical testing of traditional remedies can be seen as the most thorough testing of any medicine. The most modern drug goes through a comparatively gentle, short and less secure testing procedure. Consider briefly how these old wives' tales have travelled through history. The further back in history we look, the fewer the 'doctors' and the more often it was women who tended to the caring of the sick. They would make the diagnosis, decide on the treatment, collect the herbs and prepare any medicines. Also, the further back in history, the less leisure time women had and the more of their lives were spent in the daily necessities of feeding and clothing their family, and keeping the house operating. Only those herbal remedies that were both effective and safe would have been passed on.

Knowledge of herbs would have been passed among family members, neighbours and also to other parts of the country through travel. Mothers passed their knowledge to their daughters, who would have used and passed on only those remedies that were reliable. In this way, every household, in every generation, was a remedy testing station. Remedies have been thus tested hundreds of thousands of times and are still being tested in the same way. The same process is witnessed today. Think about the way information on new recipes, novels, films, and holiday resorts are assessed and passed on through friends and families.

The empirical testing of herbs over the centuries has not left us with much knowledge of why herbs work. However, analytical techniques and scientific experiments have increased greatly our knowledge. The active ingredients are now being identified and repeatedly experiments are confirming healing properties that have been known by generations of 'old wives'.

It may not come as any surprise that a modern, scientific herbalist uses many plants for the same healing task as would have been prescribed centuries ago. Cough remedies are an interesting example. Hyssop, elecampane, eucalyptus, sage, hoarhound, liquorice, thyme, garlic and coltsfoot are regularly used by herbalists and are found in many of the pharmaceutical preparations found in chemist shops. Almost any old herbal from any country also lists these herbs among those recommended for colds and coughs.

Medical journals and other scientific literature now publish regularly papers confirming or explaining the ancient healing properties of herbs. Garlic was shown in 1986 to be capable of lowering blood pressure, blood cholesterol, and the tendency of blood to clot in the vessels causing a thrombus. Medieval herbalists used to recommend garlic to 'purify the blood' at a time when neither the circulation of the blood nor the fact of it containing different types of cell had been discovered. Garlic has also been shown to be a powerful antiseptic and expectorant, thus justifying its popular folk use for colds and chest infections.

There may not be a plant cure for every illness as the ancient Greeks and Arabs believed, but without plants the global pharmacy would be greatly depleted and less effective. The latest drug hopes for the pharmaceutical industry, if not the human race, are all derived from plants – cancer remedies from Madagascar periwinkle (*Cantheranthus rosaceae*) and the yew tree (*Taxus baccata*), and the brain drug from the living fossil, the maidenhair tree (*Ginkgo biloba*). Meanwhile, such is faith in plants from those in the know, the pharmaceutical companies, that their search for future drugs is in the unexplored rainforests of South America not in the laboratories of universities. Our wealth of traditional remedies is an extraordinary legacy deserving of the greatest respect.

CHAPTER FOUR
Herbs and Healing

HERBS HAVE EFFECTIVE HEALING PROPERTIES, BUT HERBAL medicine is much more than the use of herbs.

Antimicrobial herbs can be used to treat chest infections; expectorants to help clear catarrh from the lungs and airways; antispasmodic herbs to relax smooth muscle; anti-inflammatory herbs to ease arthritis and skin irritations or rashes. All these uses are simply treating symptoms, and can bring great and rapid relief when needed. But this is more like the practice of orthodox Western medicine than herbal medicine.

The essence of modern herbal practice goes deeper than symptomatic treatment. The aim is to discover and then direct treatment to the underlying causes of illness. Disease is understood as being caused by a failure in the body's myriad systems of co-ordination and control, of energy, balance, and of equilibrium between the vast number of simultaneous chemical reactions and processes that are life itself. One has only to ponder the marvel of being warm blooded, *and* at a near-constant 37°C in good health, to imagine the amazing control mechanisms at work. Equal wonder surrounds the immune system, that collection of specialized blood cells and tailor-made chemicals called antibodies that protect the body from invasion by organisms as well as from foreign materials like pollen.

Any one or more symptoms may have several causes. Herbal treatment focuses on all these causes and the herbalist chooses herbs to encourage a return to normal functioning. This is important. Herbs are chosen to *stimulate* bodily function back towards the normal healthy state. Such *encouragement* of the body is in contrast to pharmaceutical drugs, which (in general) are aimed at *suppressing* bodily functions. They are used to reduce or remove symptoms and rarely to get to the original cause.

Because herbalists are treating the disordered parts of the body rather than the symptoms alone, their choices of herbs may sometimes appear puzzling. It may seem sensible to the non-herbalist to use antibiotics or anti-infectives to treat acne. But a herbalist may use a mixture of herbs chosen for their individual actions on the body (see Chapter 5): lymph and skin cleaning herbs like burdock and marigold; liver stimulants like dandelion; bowel elimination supporting herbs like yellow dock; and an immune stimulant like *Echinacea*. The aim of herbal treatment here is to stop more spots developing as well as healing those present. Two important implications follow: one person's prescription may be of no use to another and, second, without an accurate herbal diagnosis, shop-bought herbal medicines may not be successful every time. Successful herbal treatment relies on successful diagnosis and a detailed understanding of herbs.

What's more, line up ten people with the same symptoms or 'disease' before a herbalist and each may be given a totally different set of herbs. The reason is simple and important. Herbalists are concerned both with *individuals* and with how their bodies have deviated from healthy functioning. That is all there is to that important but abused term, holism.

The remainder of this chapter explains many of the important health conditions and suggests herbal approaches. Illnesses are divided into systems of the body or life stages or activities. This division is for simplicity and is *not* how a herbalist would approach the same conditions if seen in an individual patient seen at a clinic. Also the herbs suggested are only illustrative. They should not be seen as either the only useful herbs or the best choice for covering the listed conditions for an individual. One great advantage of herbal medicine is the wide range of actions available within each herb and the option to combine several herbs in a single medicine, all of which allows for patient specific prescriptions to be devised for individuals' needs.

RESPIRATORY CONDITIONS

The respiratory system includes the upper respiratory tract (nose, mouth, sinuses, throat, and trachea) and the lower respiratory tract (trachea, bronchi and lungs). The nose is designed to humidify and filter air before it is sucked literally into the lungs where vital oxygen is absorbed into the blood, and the waste product, carbon dioxide, is passed from the blood into the air for disposal on breathing out.

The whole of the respiratory tract is lined with mucous membrane. The air is sucked in by a combination of the contraction of the muscular diaphragm and the lifting up and outwards of the rib-cage. Once deep in the lungs, the gases contact millions of extremely thin air sacks called alveoli, and pass to and fro across their walls into the circulating blood.

Diseases of this system can interfere with the sucking in of air and with the absorption of air across the alveoli walls.

The **common cold** is one of the most frequently seen upper respiratory tract infections (URTIs). Despite the practice of prescribing antibiotics, which are effective only against bacteria, colds are caused by viruses. Symptoms begin typically, two to three days after contact with an infected person, with an itchy nose with watery discharge and sneezing. A sore throat, cough and change in the nasal catarrh from watery to thicker yellow or green soon follows. The infection can be followed by a bacterial infection and can travel into the lungs, middle ears or the sinuses. A cold cannot be cured, but the symptoms can be relieved and the immune system boosted to reduce the chances of future colds.

Influenza and adenovirus infections are loosely lumped under what is commonly known as the flu. This can be a serious disease. It is a virulent or strong virus that should be taken seriously. Symptoms include a sore throat with a dry cough, which may turn catarrhal after three to four days, chest pain, fever, aching limbs and, joints, and often depression. The best advice where there is fever is to stay in a warm bed, drinking plenty of fluids, attending to the symptoms. Herbalists respect mild fevers as a healthy reaction to the viral invasion and do not recommend taking aspirin to reduce the fever. A period of staying at home with little physical activity is essential for the body's defences to be mobilized. One herb, *Echinacea*, is particularly useful, sipped regularly as a linctus from the first signs of flu, it can stop the developing infection dead.

Herbs can be used to boost the immune system (*Echinacea, Astralagus*); to soothe or disinfect the throat (*Glycyrrhiza, Salvia, Myrrh*); to reduce catarrh production in the nose (*Sambucus, Solidago, Hydrastis*); to flush out sinuses to reduce build-up of catarrh (*Zingiber, Capsicum*); to clear and disinfect the lungs with expectorants (*Thymus, Inula, Marrubrium, Tussilago, Urginea, Pimpinella*).

Sinusitis is an inflammation or infection of one or both of any of four pairs of air sinuses in the front of the skull. The most commonly affected are the frontal sinuses in the bone of the forehead just above the eyes, and the maxillary sinuses, just below the eyes. When affected, the sinuses are acutely painful and are usually tender to gentle pressure. Sinus infection commonly follows a cold or other URTI. There may be a slight fever and often a slightly bloodstained mucus. Allergic rhinitis, which can affect the whole of the membrane of the nose, causing it to be inflamed and secrete excess mucus, can also cause sinusitis. Either way, mucus is trapped in the sinus chamber and the build-up of pressure causes the pain. Ignoring sinusitis may lead to a chronic state, which could be complicated with thicker mucus, which is more difficult to remove without surgical treatment.

Herbal treatment takes several routes. Any allergy would be identified and contact removed. Any tendency to regular colds or chronic catarrh, even without infections, would suggest trying to lift the immune system through diet or herbs, and ensuring the digestive system, including the bowels, was functioning properly. Catarrhal states are often related to proper diet and bowel function. Sometimes diets high in dairy food or simple carbohydrates result in catarrhal throats and a period on a healthier diet usually reduces the catarrh. Meanwhile, the sinusitis is treated by a combination of stimulating a thin mucus production to flush out the sinuses (*Capsicum, Zingiber, Armoracia*); anti-infectives to clear any infection (*Echinacea, Baptisia*, Olbas oil); membrane toning to reduce further infection, inflammation or consequent mucus (*Solidago, Glechoma, Plantago, Sambucus*).

Nasal polyps are soft, grey growths from the membrane in the nose. They may appear after chronic sinusitis or allergic rhinitis and hang into the nasal space like elongated tear drops, which reduce the passage of air. They can cause sneezing and nasal speech which is often mistaken for a cold. They tend to give chronic symptoms. Polyps are best removed surgically but can be reduced with strong astringent herbs taken in powdered form as snuff. *Quercus* and *Sanguinaria* are recommended.

Adenoiditis is unpleasant but harmless. Usually the taste of foul catarrh dripping into the back of the throat, bad breath, sore throat and an earlier infection somewhere in the URTI are clues. The back of the throat may look normal as the inflammation is higher in the throat towards the opening of the nasal passage. Treat as for colds.

Sore throats can be due to a collection of causes. Pharyngitis is an inflammation of the pharynx, which is the visible back of the mouth. Viruses or bacteria can be responsible but even tiredness or hay fever can cause a sore pharynx. Tonsillitis is more obvious, because of the sharper pain, fever, and the swollen tonsils visible on either side of the throat. Ulcerated tonsils can be particularly painful and white or yellow bacterial patches are usually visible. Quinsy, or abscesses around the tonsils, cause pain and may burst after two to four days and then heal. Lower in the throat, tracheitis and laryngitis can cause soreness but are more often recognized by a tickly cough and deepening of the voice.

Herbs for infections and to boost the immune system are used along with gargles that may be either antiseptic (*Baptisia, Echinacea*) or astringent, and which tone the membranes as well as having a disinfecting action (*Salvia, Myrrh*).

Coughs have many causes. Throat infections are obvious causes but irritants and allergens also can be responsible without any infection being involved. Smoking is a well-established and avoidable cause. Often overlooked are nervous coughs. These may be unnoticed by the cougher and are overlooked surprisingly often in clinics. Although coughs are common, they should be taken seriously and a cause found, if only to exclude serious causes like fluid on the lung or lung cancer, which should be suspected, until proven otherwise, in coughs lasting more than four weeks.

Hay fever affects at least one in ten people and there are signs it is on the increase. Pollen grains penetrate the mucosal membranes of the URT and eyes where they swell and explode, releasing starch grains, which cause the allergic reaction. The three main hay fever periods each year are due to tree pollens in the early spring, flower pollens in early summer, and grass pollens in midsummer and after. The name 'hay fever' dates from the high incidence of symptoms when hay fields were scythed and stacked by hand. Many people's symptoms appear in more than one period. Herbs like *Sambucus* and *Plantago* that tone or toughen the membranes *before* the start of the expected hay fever 'season' can stop the pollen grains entering the membranes and reduce or stop any hay fever. This treatment takes time to work and should be started four to six weeks before the hay fever season. When the attacks start, *Ephedra* and *Urtica* damp down the allergic reaction and can stop symptoms.

Asthma is a distressing and potentially dangerous condition. The bronchi, or main airways leading into the lungs, become either temporarily constricted or blocked with catarrh. Both make it harder to breathe out and the sufferer becomes short of breath, wheezes and may have a dry cough. The narrowing can be due to allergens or emotional and physical stresses. When catarrh is responsible, the breathlessness may stop suddenly when coughing dislodges the lump of catarrh. But allergy or stress-related asthma doesn't stop suddenly when the cause is removed. Some sufferers are also prey to hay fever and eczema, which are also related to the immune system. These people are described as 'atopic', meaning they have an inbuilt or genetic tendency to immune overreaction to allergens. Although asthma is on the increase (along with other disordered immune conditions) it is over-diagnosed nowadays, with patients being too readily put on steroidal inhalers.

The herbal approach focuses on tackling any allergy, causes of catarrh, or stress. Often patients already on steroids for their asthma find herbal medicine means they can drop their inhalers completely or use them rarely. Expectorant herbs and lung relaxants like *Grindelia, Lobelia, Datura* and *Ephedra* are often combined. (*Ephedra* also dampens down the immune reaction.) Relaxing herbs to relieve the effects of stress may be all that is needed in some cases. (Note: If a child or adult is already on inhalers prescribed by a doctor, these should not be stopped when herbs are tried. Always treat asthma through a qualified herbalist or doctor.)

Bronchitis is usually a sign of weakness in the lungs. It is due to an inflammation of the lining of the lungs, which leads to irritation, catarrh production, coughing, and often secondary infections. It can be acute when it usually follows a cold, or chronic after repeated acute episodes or regular lung infections of any type. The chronic state is defined as a productive cough lasting three months or more in any year. The older we become the more likely it is that chronic bronchitis will occur. Smokers are at high risk. Bronchitics end up with immovable lung infections due to the combination of accumulated thick catarrh, which bacteria relish, in the lungs and the increasing difficulty in clearing the lungs by coughing. Serious diseases can follow, especially emphysema, bronchiectasis, and pneumonia.

The essential approach removes any irritants; relieves inflammation (*Verbascum, Inula*), uses stimulating and warming expectorants (*Ipecacuanha, Solanum, Urginea, Thymus*); strengthens the lungs (*Equisetum*); and promotes efficient circulation (*Angelica, Zingiber, Capsicum*); as well as encouraging a catarrh-reducing diet.

Emphysema* and *bronchiectasis affect different parts of the lung but can be due to the same causes. Chronic bronchitis, pneumonia, or a collapsed lung can lead to either condition. In emphysema, the tiny air sacs which make up much of the lung tissue collapse together like the bubbles in a foam bath left standing. This reduces greatly the surface area and elasticity of the lung and the sufferer cannot get enough oxygen for the slightest exertion. At first it is reversible but it soon becomes progressive if not arrested. Bronchiectasis is the increased dilation of the bronchi delivering air to the lungs. It is caused by chronic infection and catarrh. A cycle of infection producing inflammation and catarrh, which harbours infection, is established. Sufferers cough continuously with loose, often frothy and mucopurulent mucous with occasional blood streaks.

It is essential to tackle the continued infections (*Echinacea, Inula, Allium, Thymus*); stimulate the immune system; clear the catarrh and strengthen the lungs much as in the approach to bronchitis.

Pneumonia is the inflammation of the lungs due to various bacteria or to viruses. The lungs can also be inflamed because of allergic reactions or dust, when the condition is called pneumonitis or alveolitis. Sometimes the breathing in of vomit or a collapse of the lungs' defence mechanisms during periods of unconsciousness cause aspiration pneumonias. Infective types are divided into lobar (if the lung tissue itself is affected) and bronchopneumonia (when only the tubes, or bronchi, leading into the lungs are involved). Aspiration pneumonia results from breathing vomit or other irritating fluids into the lungs.

Pneumonia is always potentially serious. Infections elsewhere, especially in the URT, can descend into the lungs causing pneumonias. This is a common cause of death among the elderly, particularly after surgery or any other illness or event that weakens them.

Pneumonia is difficult to diagnose accurately but any persistent cough with fever, rusty-coloured catarrh being coughed up, or chest pain on coughing should be suspect immediately.

Where bacterial infection is confirmed, antibiotics should be taken, if recommended by a doctor, as this is the more serious form of the disease. Herbs still have an important role. Infective pneumonias usually strike generally weakened people or people with a history of lung infections. Treatment would consider first the infection or other cause of inflammation (e.g. *Echinacea, Inula, Plantago, Equisetum, Verbascum*). Anticatarrhals are usually necessary to help clear the copious catarrh produced (e.g. *Marrubrium, Urginea, Hyssopus, Thymus*). As the immediate condition subsides, herbs to strengthen the immune system and lung tissue would follow together with a general rehabilitation programme aimed at returning the strength of the whole body (e.g. *Glycyrrhiza, Elutherococcus, Berberis*).

Pleurisy may follow serious infections like pneumonia. It is the inflammation of the thin membranes that separate the lungs from the chest wall. The symptoms are pain on breathing in or on coughing. Treat as for lung infections.

Pleural effusion is fluid between the lungs and chest wall. The only symptoms may be a cough and difficulty breathing because the fluid presses against the lungs making it difficult for them to fill completely. Many conditions can lead to an effusion. The herbalist would treat the underlying condition.

Beware of any of the following symptoms, which may indicate conditions that should be treated by a doctor or herbalist:

- coughing of blood or blood-streaked or rusty sputum

- any fever that lasts more than four days

- chest pain on breathing

- unexplained difficulty in breathing

- any change in colouring around the mouth or tongue towards blueness

EARS AND EYES

The ears and eyes are vital and sensitive organs that keep us in touch with the world around us. Both are delicate and suffer from common annoying conditions. The eye is well designed to look after itself but the ear is an organ better designed for operating in a protective glass case than in the real world. The external canal invites the accumulation of dirt, water and its own protective wax, all of which can lead to infections and temporary deafness. The middle ear on each side of the head is connected to the throat by a tube up which can pass infected catarrh from the URT or water during swimming and scuba diving, causing infections in an isolated pocket within the ear.

Otitis externa means inflammation or infection of the external canal leading to the eardrum. Dust can carry bacteria; water trapped in the canal can cause softening of skin which allows bacterial infections; excess wax can block the canal leading to infection. Eczema and boils are common in the canal. After examining the ear canal, the immediate cause can be identified and treated. Wax can be softened with drops of *Hypericum* or mullein oil. As it clears use anti-inflammation drops containing anti-microbial or tissue-healing herbs (*Symphytum, Hypericum, Allium, Verbascum, Stellaria, Calendula*). Boils in the canal can be treated with *Calendula* oil and eczema with *Calendula* cream.

Otitis media involves the middle ear which houses the three small bones that transmit the sound vibrations from the eardrum to the inner ear and the special nerves of hearing. The middle ear is an air filled space, lined with mucous membrane and joined to the upper throat by two thin tubes. Infected catarrh or water can be blown up these tubes by coughing or nose blowing and thus infect the lining of the middle ear. Once the membrane is infected or inflamed, it too secretes mucus which can both block the exit tubes and cause increased pressure within the inner ear. The result can be deafness and earache. Young children are especially susceptible because their eustachian tubes are shorter and they tend to have more catarrhal conditions in the head than adults. Glue ear is a particularly bad case of catarrhal otitis media. Sometimes the eardrum can perforate and there can be a discharge of pus or mucus into the ear canal. Perforation of the eardrum is common. It usually heals, especially in children but the hole can remain unhealed, leaving an easy entry for infections into the middle ear.

Herbal treatment would tackle the infections plus any other causes of excess catarrh in the ear, diet for example, then look to membrane-toning herbs to dry and stem future production of catarrh (*Solidago, Glechoma, Plantago, Hydrastis, Sambucus*).

Deafness has many causes. Defects in the ear at birth, infections like meningitis or mumps, excess loud noise at work, or simple loss of efficiency of the moving parts with old age should not be overlooked. But there are some common causes of temporary deafness with simple solutions. Ear canals blocked with wax cause varying degrees of deafness. The solution can be softening the wax with *Hypericum* oil drops and allowing the softened wax to drain away. Syringing may be necessary but should be avoided if possible. Excess catarrh in the middle ear, with or without infection, can damp the movements of the drum and little bones of the ear, thus making hearing faint and muffled. Anticatarrhal treatments above are effective.

Tinnitus is annoying. Constant ringing, 'whooshing', or whistling sounds in the ears are distracting. Causes are not always fully understood but it is clear that catarrh in the middle ear can cause it, as can reduced circulation around the auditory nerve in the structures of the inner ear. Herbal treatments for excess catarrh as above and with circulatory remedies (*Ginkgo, Zanthoxylum, Zingiber*) can be very effective. Any circulatory problem needs careful diagnosis and appropriate treatment so it is best to plan such treatment through a herbalist.

Many eye conditions need specialist treatment because they involve the inner workings of the eye. However, superficial conditions can be treated safely and easily with herbs.

Conjunctivitis is well known as the cause of pink eyes, grittiness and the yellow discharge that can stick the eyelids together during sleep. It is due to an inflammation of the thin membrane covering the white cornea of the eyes. Bacteria are usually responsible but it is also caused by allergic reactions. Sometimes physical damage to the eye surface from scratches or dust precipitate infections. Effective treatment with eyewashes of *Calendula* or *Euphrasia* help. Preventive measures, keeping away from dusty environments and washing thoroughly all personal towels and bed linen, reduce the chance of reinfections.

Blepharitis is a form of eczema or seborrhoea of the eyelids. It may be allergic and should be treated as for eczema. Relieve the scaling and redness with *Calendula* or *Matricaria* creams.

Sties are painful abscesses at the base of the eyelashes. They are caused by bacteria but unlike boils elsewhere on the body are not necessarily associated with a run-down immune system or poor hygiene and diet. They may be spread from bacteria in the nose through nose picking, or from other sites of bacterial infection. Treat with hot compresses (*Matricaria* flowers, *Althaea* leaves) which help draw out the infection and lead to a bursting of the abscess and its healing. Sties may reoccur.

DIGESTIVE SYSTEM

The human body is like a doughnut. If it were elastic and held at the mouth and anus ends before stretching the full length of the intestine (22 feet), it would be possible to look in the mouth and see light out of the anus. The digestive tract is like a 22-foot long tube (or hole through the doughnut) running from the mouth to the anus. Most of it is stuffed loosely into a 12-inch high trunk, the abdomen. The lining of the doughnut's hole or the digestive tract is a specialized form of the skin that covers the outside of the doughnut.

As the outer skin varies in design for different functions, so the lining of the digestive tract also changes for different functions along its length. Special glands in the mouth secrete saliva to moisten and partially digest food before swallowing. The stomach has special secreting cells whereas the colon has special water-absorbing cells and muscles to move waste material along. If the digestive tract is visualized as a skin-covered muscular tube with parts that secrete and parts that absorb, many of its diseases can be easily understood.

Health depends on all the functions of the digestive tract working efficiently. It has to break up and moisten food, cover it in digestive acids and enzymes, then move the food into the intestine where more enzymes and digestive chemicals are added before the absorption of water and nutrients starts. Waste material from the blood is injected into the intestine as bile for elimination and, as the nutrients are absorbed from the digested food, the waste leftovers have to be moved through to the end of the intestine and passed out of the body. Simple and impressive!

Mouth ulcers (Aphthous ulcers) are painful white circles inside the mouth. They are usually 1-3mm across and are slightly sunken. The cause is unknown but they are associated with a run-down immune system and poor eating habits. They usually come in clusters and are a reliable sign that some body maintenance is needed or other illness will surely follow.

While attention to general health is being organized, the most effective treatment is to paint undiluted tincture of myrrh (*Commiphora*) on isolated ulcers. Ulcers go in twenty-four to forty-eight hours. If there are several around the mouth or they keep appearing, use diluted myrrh tincture as a mouthwash.

Gingivitis is more annoying than serious but it can lead to serious infections in the mouth that damage teeth. Poor cleaning of teeth or persistent infections in the mouth inflame the gums. Gums may bleed, especially on brushing, which may be the first sign of gum problems. A refresher course on dental hygiene is advised.

Mouthwashes with gentle herbal astringents (*Salvia, Quercus, Potentilla*) help reduce the inflammation. A mouthwash with myrrh or *Echinacea* may be necessary if the infection has taken hold within the gums.

Candidiasis (Moniliasis or oral thrush) is an overgrowth of the natural gut-inhabiting fungus, *Candida albicans*, due to an impaired immune system. Antibiotics, debilitation from other illnesses, stress of any type, and poor eating habits can be involved. The organism is a fungus that normally lives on and in the body. When rampant in the mouth there are white blotches on the cheeks or tongue that can be scraped off. Treatment with herbs is simple but this is a typical condition that will return and return until the underlying causes are tackled. If in doubt check with a herbalist.

Herbs to remove the fungus from the mouth include *Calendula, Melaleuca, Echinacea, Thymus*. Treatment might also address the immune system (*Echinacea, Elutherococcus*); the liver (*Berberis, Taraxacum, Hydrastis*); and look to the effects of stress on the body's systems (*Glycyrrhiza, Elutherococcus, Verbena, Jateorrhiza, Chelone*).

Oesophagitis announces itself with burning pain behind the breast bone or sternum. The oesophagus is the tube channelling food from the mouth to the stomach. Between it and the stomach is a valve to stop the stomach's contents going back up the oesophagus. When this valve fails or when there is a hiatus hernia, stomach contents and acids are forced upwards. Symptoms are worse on lying down, bending over, or after excessively large meals. It burns because the oesophagus is not designed to have stomach acids washing its walls. Oesophagitis can also be caused by either swallowing irritating liquids or infections. If untreated, ulceration can result.

Occasionally surgery is needed but early action can remove the problem. Kind handling of the stomach often removes symptoms. Avoidance of chocolate, coffee and alcohol helps as does eating small meals often. The pain can be relieved with herbal demulcents (*Althaea, Symphytum, Glycyrrhiza, Ulmus*); inflammation of the tissues healed with anti-inflammatories (*Matricaria, Filipendula*); and excess acidity (*Filipendula, Acorus*).

Gastritis differs from the milder stomach complaint loosely called indigestion in that vomiting is common. Infections or any irritant in food can cause it. Infections are commonly announced by a fever, but not always. Alcohol is a potent irritant of the stomach and excessive drinkers can expect chronic gastritis. The best attack is through removing the dubious food, identifying the cause and nature of any infection, and soothing the irritated stomach.

Chronic gastritis can also be caused by stress and emotional tension. This is called a 'functional' condition and is associated with indigestion, peptic ulcers, and irritable bowel syndrome. Liver and gall bladder disease or hepatitis, not to forget the most popular painkiller, aspirin, can produce symptoms of gastritis, so careful diagnosis is advised.

Relaxing herbs (*Tilia, Matricaria, Melissa*) should be prescribed as necessary, with soothing stomach herbs (*Filipendula, Comfrey, Glycyrrhiza, Ulmus*) to bring quick relief. Food-poisoning bacteria can be treated with crushed fresh garlic or *Thymus*. Attend also to any other contributing factor to avoid recurrences.

Peptic ulcer is a catch-all for ulcers in the stomach as well as the first part of the small intestine, the duodenum, and for severe gastritis that produces the same symptoms. Ulcer sufferers know the sharp, localized pain at the base of the sternum, which is relieved by eating or taking antacids. It is rarely there all the time, but in bouts either soon after eating (stomach ulcer) or several hours later (duodenal ulcer). A barium X-ray or endoscope examination are the only ways of making a positive diagnosis.

There is uncertainty over the causes. It seems that excess acidity is essential for ulceration to start but the actual cause is a mystery. Recent research suggests that invasion of the stomach wall by a bacterium, *Helicobacter pylori*, may cause the increased acid production. But stress, irregular eating and stomach wall irritants may all play a part.

Herbs have been shown to speed healing of ulcers. German doctors use the excellent anti-inflammatory and antibacterial, Chamomile tea. It is drunk each morning on an empty stomach before the patient lies on the floor for one hour. Every fifteen minutes the patient rolls over ninety degrees ensuring that every square centimetre of the stomach wall is bathed in the tea. Less athletic herbal treatment uses *Glycyrrhiza, Symphytum*, and *Filipendula* which protect the ulcer and promote its healing. A dramatic reassessment of lifestyle is usually necessary as well.

Dyspepsia or indigestion is a common complaint. Often it is due to rapid eating of large meals that are too fatty, rich or spicy. Stress is usually part of the picture. Symptoms include discomfort around the stomach, nausea, wind, colic, and regurgitation of stomach acid into the back of the mouth.

Herbalists attend to eating habits if necessary and can use acidity-lowering herbs (*Filipendula*); carminatives, which relax the gut wall and relieve colic and wind (*Pimpinella, Foeniculum, Mentha, Matricaria, Cardamom, Zingiber*); or digestive stimulants if sluggish digestion is involved (*Acorus, Chelone, Jateorrhiza, Artemesia*).

Anorexia or poor appetite can be worrying long before weight loss becomes life threatening. Many of the body's essential nutrients cannot be stored in the body so must be eaten regularly. Severe psychological disorder is behind anorexia nervosa and appropriate action is necessary. However, many people suffer 'going off their food' for short periods. Many minor conditions from flu to anxiety can cause loss of appetite but liver problems, glandular fever and many drugs are also culprits.

Simple herbal digestive stimulants are useful to encourage digestive 'tone' and function. Bitter herbs are traditional digestive 'kick–starts' (*Gentiana, Centaury, Artemesia, Acorus, Jateorrhiza, Taraxacum*).

Diarrhoea and constipation are opposite ends of a scale of healthy bowel function, a concept too little discussed and thus misunderstood. It is not necessary to have a daily bowel motion. There is a wide range of 'normality' among individuals. Some go two or three times a day whereas others may go only every second day. The important word is 'regularity' not frequency. Ideal consistency should not be a large 'well formed' stool but a thin ribbon the consistency of cake icing being squeezed from an icing bag. It should pass effortlessly. Too firm a stool and the colon has to work too hard moving it around, and the bowel has to push too much to release it from the body. Hard stools invite diverticulitis, piles and fissures.

Constipation may be caused by stress or poor diet. The bowel can lose tone and stop moving the waste material along or can become spastic when the muscular walls contract and stay tight, disrupting the rhythmical peristaltic action that normally moves the waste along.

Correct diagnosis is important. A toneless bowel may benefit from stimulation but one already in spasm could be made worse by using stimulant laxatives.

Before reaching for laxatives, finding the cause is important. Often simply correcting diet or attending to stress is all that is needed. Never be confident that a diet has enough dietary fibre, or bulk, without checking with a dietician, herbalist or in a suitable book. But even if the foods in the diet are rich in bulk, enough food has to be eaten to supply sufficient bulk for the bowel to work on. Too little food is a common cause of constipation in the elderly, the sick, the anxious and depressed, or in dieters.

The best herbal laxative is food. Increasing the am
fibre foods like dried apricots, pulses, whole cereals an
etables may be enough. Sometimes gentle stimulation o
with liver herbs is sufficient as bile encourages normal rh   ....ical
movements of the bowel. Efficient bulking laxatives are psyllium
husks (*Plantago ovata*) and crushed linseed. Lactulose is an osmotic
laxative which holds water in the bowel so a dry stool cannot be
formed. Stimulant laxatives irritate the lining of the bowel, encouraging peristalsis to pass the irritating chemical quickly (*Cascara,
Cassia*). These usually work six to eight hours after taking the laxative.

Diarrhoea can be due to infections, food poisoning, and intolerances, or stress. Simple change of diet or water can upset the
digestive system and a few bouts of diarrhoea within twenty-four
to forty-eight hours can result. Infections should be identified if
possible from a stool sample sent to a laboratory. Drugs may be
responsible so check for any side effects of current medication.
Diarrhoea should always be investigated if it lasts more than forty-
eight hours as causes like inflammatory bowel disease, pancreatic
disease, and bowel cancers could be responsible.

Simple diarrhoea can be helped with astringent herbs that calm
the lining of the bowel (*Potentilla, Geum, Agrimonia, Quercus*).
When diarrhoea persists always take plenty of fluids.

Irritable bowel syndrome or IBS is said to affect 40 per cent of
Western populations. Symptoms include alternating loose stools
and constipation, bloating, abdominal pain or discomfort. Some
people tend to longer periods of diarrhoea and they often pass
mucus as well. This is not really a disease but a collection of symptoms and can have many causes. Herbal experience suggests that as
many as 80 per cent of sufferers have emotional stress regularly in
their lives and that many of the remainder may have food intolerances, mild inflammation of the bowel or all three.

Contrary to common opinion, this is not a condition that must
be tolerated. Most people can find significant or complete relief
with herbs. Careful history taking will identify stress or intolerance

actors, which must be addressed. Herbal medication can help with antispasmodics (*Viburnum, Valeriana, Dioscorea, Melissa*) to calm the bowel or toning herbs (*Agrimonia, Filipendula*). Any underlying stress must be tackled.

Diverticulitis can be painful and distressing. It is known as right-sided appendicitis because of the character of the pain. When the lower bowel is under pressure from a life of trying to pass over-hard stools, small pockets of the gut wall can balloon outwards, forming small pouches. If these become infected or inflamed, they can produce pain, bleeding and diarrhoea.

Improving the diet is essential. A soft stool will stop the condition worsening and can stop recurrences once the inflammation is treated. Use herbs to relax the bowel, heal the inflammation and tone the wall (*Agrimonia, Symphytum, Dioscorea, Matricaria, Filipendula*).

Inflammatory bowel diseases include Crohn's disease and ulcerative colitis. Inflammation and ulceration of the intestine, usually in patches, leads to pain, poor absorption of nutrients, diarrhoea and sometimes passing blood, pus or mucus in the stools. Several different conditions are included. Causes are largely unknown but it is thought that stress, infection and possibly food allergies may be involved. These conditions are diagnosed after barium X-rays and internal examinations.

Herbal treatment can help heal the inflammation if caught early, using mucilaginous, astringent and adrenal stimulating herbs (*Symphytum, Agrimonia, Plantago, Glycyrrhiza, Matricaria*).

Jaundice and liver disease are of great significance to herbalists who recognize the importance of efficient liver function to almost everything else that happens in the body. An inefficient or malfunctioning liver can be behind so many common illnesses. Jaundice is due to the presence of bilirubin, a natural breakdown product of blood pigment. Excess bilirubin may be due to a rapid and abnormal breakdown of red blood cells or, more usually, to either an interference with liver function or a blockage stopping bile leaving the liver where it is produced. Both infections and many pharmaceutical drugs can cause liver inflammation and jaundice. Medical diagnosis is essential before treatment. Most jaundice is due to minor and reversible conditions, but diseases like cirrhosis or cancers in the liver may be involved.

Herbs can help with liver damage (*Cardus, Cynara*) or inflammation (*Taraxacum, Chelidonium*) as well as promoting a healthy liver function through appropriate bitters (*Gentiana, Berberis, Centaurea*). Careful checking of any recent medication may identify drug causes of jaundice.

Gall-bladder disease is surprisingly common. Many people have gallstones even though they may have no symptoms now or in the future. Inflammation of the gall bladder is common and gives symptoms of discomfort under the right ribs, indigestion, intolerance of fatty foods and flatulence. Given that this organ stores bile, which is a toxic mixture of processed waste products from the liver awaiting dumping into the intestine for disposal, is it any wonder it sometimes gets inflamed?

Diet can reduce the chances of stones occurring or of existing stones getting worse. There is some evidence that large amounts of olive oil and lemon juice drunk over one to two days can expel small stones. Herbalists tackle the tendency to form stones by increasing the production and flow of bile from the liver (choleretic), thus diluting the bile and reducing the chances of stones forming (*Berberis, Rosmarinus, Acorus, Hydrastis, Chelone, Taraxacum*). Simple bitter and aromatic herbs help by stimulating digestive processes and thus the emptying of the gall bladder (cholagogue) into the intestine (*Gentiana, Centaurea, Artemesia*). Many herbs are both choleretic and cholagogue and the herbalist would normally encourage both functions. Inflammation of the gall bladder is treated with *Chelidonium*.

Pancreatitis is serious and provides excruciating pain, which all sufferers remember clearly. Gall-bladder disease, infections elsewhere, alcoholism, or drugs (steroids and diuretics) are common causes of inflammation within the pancreas due to excess production of pancreatic enzymes. These are designed to digest proteins in the intestine but end up digesting those of the pancreatic tissue and other organs of the body. Symptoms include pain centred around the stomach and radiating to the back, nausea and vomiting, profound shock and rapid heartbeat.

There can also be chronic pancreatitis where a low level of irritation exists. This is made worse by alcohol. Herbs can do little for the acute crisis, but can help chronic cases by keeping the liver and gall bladder functioning healthily and reducing gravel or stone build-up. Choice as for jaundice above.

Piles are really varicose veins in the rectum. Under pressure from bearing down to pass large, hard stools, veins are stretched. Pregnant women also suffer from piles. They are painful and may bleed.

Herbal treatment looks to the bowel function as well as the symptoms. Veins can be 'toned' (*Aesculus, Fagopyrum*) to reduce stretching and ballooning. The bleeding can be reduced by applying astringents directly to the piles (*Quercus, Hamamelis, Achillea, Potentilla*).

Beware of any of the following symptoms, which may indicate conditions that should be treated by a doctor or herbalist:

- pain in centre of chest, which may not be due to dyspepsia

- feeling of lumps or constriction behind sternum or breastbone

- passing bloody or black stools

- vomiting blood

- rapid loss of weight

- change in bowel habit (mucus or looseness)

- 'indigestion' pain that lasts three or more days

HEART AND CIRCULATION

The circulation of blood takes nutrients and oxygen to every living cell in the body and carries away waste materials of cellular activities and of carbon dioxide for processing and disposal. Important additional functions include carrying nutrients from the intestine, being an effective delivery system for the body's chemical control mechanism (hormones) and for carrying the protective immune system in the form of special blood cells and proteins. Not only must the blood be healthy, but the pump and all the blood vessels must be able to deliver the blood efficiently.

The blood travels away from the pumping heart in arteries and returns through veins. The large arteries branch and narrow progressively into arterioles and finally into capillaries barely wide enough for single red blood cells to pass through. Hardening (arteriosclerosis) or 'furring' (atherosclerosis) of blood vessels restricts flow, especially in peripheral parts of the body. This, combined with any 'thickening' of the blood which makes it more difficult for it to flow through narrow vessels, can stop or reduce greatly the blood supply. This mixture of factors is behind many heart attacks, which occur when vessels supplying part of the heart muscle cannot carry enough oxygen to the heart and part of the muscle falters or stops.

It often surprises people that blood vessels are elastic and their diameter is constantly changing to suit the need for a changing volume of blood flow or to control the pressure of the flowing blood. The autonomic nervous system controls this diameter in response to changes in body temperature, demand for blood in muscles, changes in blood pressure, and even emotional stress. If this control goes wrong, an excess blood pressure can result, or there might be shortage of blood flow to limbs (e.g. Raynaud's syndrome). Sudden changes in the distribution of blood can lead to dizziness or fainting and are called vasovagal attacks, after the vagus nerve which is one of the main blood-flow controlling nerves. The best known effect of elastic blood vessels is varicose veins. **Warning**: Many conditions affecting the heart, blood and circulation are potentially serious and should be treated only through a doctor or herbalist.

High blood pressure or hypertension is rare in the Third World but common in industrial societies where, from the age of twenty-five, blood pressures tend to creep upwards. A slightly raised pressure is not healthy but should not cause concern unless the diastolic (or lower reading) pressure is persistently over one hundred. Doctors disagree over when a raised blood pressure should be treated.

Too high a blood pressure can cause heart failure, heart attacks or strokes. Headaches or dizziness may suggest a raised pressure but most people have no symptoms, even with very high pressures. It is simple to measure and everyone should have their blood pressure measured regularly.

Causes may be stress, obesity, diet, kidney malfunction or hormone changes. No cause is found in over 90 per cent of cases, when the condition is given the odd name of 'essential hypertension'.

It used to be said once a patient was put on drugs to lower blood pressure, they were on them for life. This is not necessarily true. Many cases of raised pressure may benefit from drugs to reduce risk of complications. But it is often possible to return the pressure to safe or normal levels by lifestyle changes. Controlling weight, taking exercise, correcting the diet, and reducing stress should be explored as relevant.

Herbalists look for all possible causes and can treat anxiety or its effects on the heart (*Valeriana, Melissa, Tilia, Leonurus, Crateagus*); reduce water retention with diuretics (*Taraxacum, Parietaria*); and reduce blood pressure through increasing the volume of blood in the peripheral arteries (*Achillea, Tilia*). Help with weight, diet, exercise and stress management are considered where relevant. Lower than normal blood pressure is not often of health significance, but where necessary *Sarothamnus* will raise a low blood pressure.

Vasovagal attacks The blood pressure and output of the heart are controlled by a network of sensitive and finely tuned mechanisms. The vagus nerve is part of the parasympathetic half of the autonomic (or automatic) nervous system. It dilates the blood vessels, which is the opposite action to the flight and fight response of stress, and slows the heartbeat. When this happens, either suddenly due to emotional stress or with the system out of control, there can be a brief lowering of blood pressure, a drop in blood supply to the brain, and dizziness or fainting follows. The effects are usually temporary and can be relieved by moderating the response to stress or, with herbs, by relaxing the body and relieving the anxiety responses (*Valeriana, Verbena, Melissa, Scutellaria*).

Angina is a sign that the heart is under stress. Typical symptoms of stabbing pains in the chest, or even in the jaw or down the left arm, come on with exercise or emotional stress. When the trigger is removed, the pain goes after five minutes or so. Angina itself is not serious. It is only a symptom, but it is both painful and frightening. It should be reported to a doctor for a thorough heart check by a cardiologist.

Herbal approaches improve the circulation to the heart muscle (*Crateagus, Ammi*) and may also help with reducing the effect of stress on the patient (*Leonurus, Valeriana, Verbena*). Your doctor should always be notified of herbal treatment.

Heart failure is common after many diseases of the circulation that place greater strain or demand on the heart: arteriosclerosis, heart attacks, valve diseases, diseases that cause obstruction in the lungs, and a hyperactive thyroid gland. Contrary to the name, the heart doesn't stop, but it finds it progressively harder to pump the blood needed by the body. In short, it fails to deliver enough blood most of the time. The problem may affect either the left or right side of the heart, or both. Symptoms are shortage of breath, cough, congested and swollen liver, swelling of the ankles and around the lower spine. Treatment is well advised but in mild degrees of 'failure' patients can live many years with only restricted activity to remind them of their problem.

Treatment is directed at the causes, which may include lung disease like emphysema or bronchitis, thyroid problems, anaemia, and diseases of the arteries. Appropriate herbal treatment should follow. For the heart itself, *Convallaria* or lily of the valley is as useful as foxglove extract which is used in hospitals as the drug digoxin. The foxglove drug is very toxic, presenting extra dangers, but *Convallaria* is as effective and safer. Often simply encouraging the heart to pump more effectively makes the kidney work properly and ankle swelling disappears. Where there is water retention, diuretics may be added to the prescription to encourage water loss through the kidneys (*Taraxacum, Ononis, Betula*). **Warning**: Never treat heart failure without consulting a doctor or herbalist.

Heart attacks remain a serious cause of early death and illness in industrial countries despite some reductions since the 1960s. This is one of the few important diseases that afflict men more than women, at least until the age of seventy. There is no room for complacency. Death is often the first evidence of the diseased arteries supplying the heart muscle. Prevention is best. Removing or reducing risk factors like smoking, inactivity, raised blood cholesterols, obesity, excessive alcohol, and high blood pressure are essential steps. There is a genetic component but that cannot explain the disease, although it increases the chances of members of the same family having the disease. The more evidence of a family history, the more reason to reduce other risk factors.

Herbalists are health promoters in their approach to all illness. They seek to improve the functioning of the whole body and thus reduce disease. They can advise on the reduction of heart disease risk factors, especially diet. In general, raised dietary fat, especially all saturated fats, excess sugar and salt, together with a shortage of dietary fibre, are the main culprits. Healthy eating is not boring eating. Most people find their eating pleasure is improved, while their chances of having a long list of diet-related illness is dramatically reduced.

Strokes are due to damage to part of the brain. The culprits are either a blood clot causing a blockage in a blood vessel serving the brain or blood leaking from a blood vessel into the brain tissue. Symptoms depend on where in the brain the damage occurs and how widespread it is.

Herbalists can help with both recovery and preventing further strokes. Circulation-improving herbs (*Ginkgo, Melilotus, Aesculus, Achillea*) together with herbal treatment of any raised blood pressure, help with relaxing, and diet improvements may be considered.

Varicose veins are common and more unsightly than a health hazard. The problem is a swelling or ballooning of the vein walls so that the internal valves no longer work. Gravitational pressure on the column of blood in veins increases and pushes the walls out further. Sometimes there may be inflammation of the veins as well and this can lead to clotting, which could be serious. Varicose veins are more common among women than men, and tend to run in families.

Herbalists treat varicose veins by relieving inflammation and strengthening or toning the vascular walls (*Aesculus, Ruta, Melilotus, Fagopyrum*), which can arrest the condition but not reverse it. Circulatory support may be added with *Achillea* and *Tilia*. External creams of *Calendula, Juniperus* and *Aesculus* help with local inflammation and pain.

Temporal arteritis is an unexplained inflammation of the arteries passing over the temples. There is usually headache and the arteries are tender. Often there are signs of rheumatic disease affecting the muscles or joints, or of inflammation elsewhere in the circulatory system. It should be taken seriously as it can lead to blindness.

After careful checking for signs of inflammation elsewhere, herbalists use anti-inflammatory herbs (*Aesculus, Salix, Guaiacum, Glycyrrhiza*) along with rheumatic herbs (*Harpogophytum, Salix, Apium, Tanacetum*).

Raynaud's syndrome is due to an unexplained spasm of the arteries in the fingers or toes in response to cold. Fingers go white, then blue and numb.

Herbal treatment can be internal or external only. The aim is to combine antispasmodics to relax the arterial spasm with herbs that stimulate the flow of blood to the hands and feet (*Viburnum, Ginkgo, Achillea, Zingiber*). Because the arteries of the hands and feet are close to the skin, topical creams are an ideal way of delivering the medicine. Relaxing and heating creams can be rubbed into the affected parts before they are exposed to cold (*Viburnum, Cinnamomum, Cajaput, Syzygium, Melaleuca*).

Chilblains are painful red swellings on hands and feet caused by poor circulation. Sufferers usually have cold hands and feet. It is the application of heat to tightly constricted blood vessels that causes the irritation leading to the chilblain.

The best herbal treatment is the use of circulatory stimulants directed at the peripheral areas (*Achillea, Zingiber*), together with plenty of exercise to stimulate circulation. Affected areas should be warmed from inside the body rather than by applying external heat via a fire or radiator.

Varicose ulcers are a frustrating infliction on the elderly. They tend to follow the slightest bruise or injury below the knees on people with poor circulation, especially in the legs. These ulcers are difficult to heal and are often left for too long before presenting them for treatment. Because a healthy blood supply is essential for the healing of any wound, the reduced flow to the legs explains both the appearance of the ulcer and why it usually takes so long to heal.

Herbalists recognize the role of circulation and try to increase the flow to the legs as well as treating the infection itself. Circulation herbs (*Aesculus, Zanthoxylum, Achillea, Capsicum*) are used internally. The ulcer is washed with infusions of anti-infectives (*Thymus, Calendula, Quercus, Myrrh*), while the outer inflamed areas around the ulcer itself have healing creams applied (*Symphytum, Aesculus, Calendula*). Exercise to the feet and legs is important. This needn't require walking but only simple exercises that can be done while in a chair or even a bed. Anyone with circulation problems in the legs should not smoke, should keep intake of alcohol to a minimum, and should make sure the diet is healthy.

Beware of any of the following symptoms, which may indicate conditions that should be treated by a doctor or herbalist:

- pain in the chest, jaw or down the left arm

- persistent headaches or dizzy spells

- shortage of breath on mild exercise

- swollen ankles at the end of the day

- chronic low energy or rapid heart beat

- very cold, pale or blue feet or hands

- any slow-healing wound below the knee in an elderly person

MUSCULO-SKELETAL SYSTEM

The bony skeleton provides protection for internal organs, gives recognizable form to the body, and, together with the skeletal muscles, is the means of moving and of manipulating objects.

Bone tissue is not only for structural support. Inside the bone is marrow, which plays an important part in the regeneration of blood cells. The bone itself is an enormous reservoir of minerals, which are being continually released into the blood and reabsorbed according to need and dietary intake. Healthy bone adjusts its structure and thickness to the demands placed on it and to dietary adequacy. The less physical activity taken, the more the bones become thin and more honeycombed in structure, making them brittle and weak.

Muscles also develop to meet physical need. The more work is demanded of a group of muscles, the more they are developed and are taut or toned. Part of health maintenance is exercising all the body's muscle groups for all-round fitness. Fit muscles are less likely to 'tear' or be strained by unaccustomed exertion.

There are many diseases of the structure and growth of bone and muscle (e.g. Paget's disease, muscular dystrophy, ankylosing spondylitis, osteoporosis) that require specialist diagnosis and treatment. But many common enough conditions are susceptible to herbal treatment.

Strains and sprains are the commonest injury to this system. Strained muscles are due to either sudden or excess work being asked of muscle. This causes tearing or stretching of the fibres in the body of the muscle. Afterwards there is sharp pain on actively contracting the muscle, tenderness over the injured area, swelling and, possibly, visible bruising. Much back pain is due to simple muscle strain, often from something so common as bending over the rim of a car boot to place the shopping inside.

Sprains are tears or stretches to the strong fibrous ligaments that surround the joints and keep them firmly together. A sprained ankle from a slight stumble that bends the ankle joint too far outwards is common enough. Symptoms are swelling, pain and sometimes bruising.

Treat both with ice packs to remove any swelling. If there is no swelling (or when it has been reduced), then topical creams with anti-inflammatories (*Gaultheria*), warming herbs to bring healing blood into the area (*Camphora, Syzygium, Rosmarinus*), tissue healing herbs (*Symphytum*), blood-dispersant herbs where there is bruising (*Arnica*), and muscle relaxants if there is any protective muscle spasm around the injury (*Viburnum, Lavandula*). A very old and effective recipe for sprains and strains includes the leaves of *Sambucus, Artemesia vulgaris, Plantago*, and *Glechoma*. Never immobilize the injured part but keep it moving with gentle exercises without weight or strain.

Cramps can plague equally the fittest athlete and the most proficient 'couch potato'. Cramps are strong spasms in muscle.

Most cramp is due to waste product (lactic acid) accumulating in main muscles during energetic physical activity like running or playing football. They can also occur in hot, sweaty conditions when people have not had time to acclimatize. Normally, after two weeks in a hot country or doing sweaty jobs, the body adapts to the high sweat loss and retains much of the salt that would otherwise be lost in sweat. People who suffer from leg or foot cramps regularly under conditions where they do not sweat much may be short of sodium (salt) but more likely calcium or potassium.

Cramps may also be due to vascular problems in the legs causing shortage of blood supply. Internal circulation stimulants (*Zanthoxylum, Capsicum, Armoracia, Galangal, Angelica*) and creams containing muscle relaxants (*Viburnum, Lavandula*) can reduce frequency. Although deficiencies of calcium and potassium are uncommon, it is worth checking the diet with a herbalist or dietician.

Tennis elbow and golfer's elbow are related painful problems affecting the tendons on the outside and inside of the elbow respectively. Rest assured that neither golf nor tennis must be played to become a sufferer. Both are due to persistent stress on the muscle attachments (tendons) that join the muscle to the inside or outside of the elbow joint. Golfer's elbow may be triggered by actions similar to using a screwdriver whereas tennis elbow is more likely from actions that flex and straighten the wrist.

Herbal treatment includes avoiding habitual strenuous activity with the affected arm but not resting the arm completely. Gentle exercise that keeps the muscles of the forearm in use and flexes the elbow will help healing. Hot compresses together with anti-inflammatory creams (*Gaultheria*), laced with circulation stimulating herbs (*Camphora, Cajaput, Rosmarinus*), and tissue healers (*Symphytum*) used patiently over one to three months will ensure healing.

Tensosynovitis is a common cause of pain in the hands and wrists, occasionally in the feet as well. Inflammation of the lining of muscle tendons after persistent use is the main cause. Sometimes an infection may be the cause. Treat with resting the limb and using the same herbal treatments as for tennis elbow.

Frozen shoulder usually means just that. There is pain on movement and movement is difficult because of stiffness of the shoulder joint. The problem is due to inflammation within the joint but there is no agreed explanation. Some theories suggest it is associated with disease elsewhere in the body, others with some stressful use of the shoulder or even because of not enough use.

Whatever the cause, the treatment is conservative. Always try to keep the shoulder moving by not using a sling and doing regular light exercises putting the shoulder through the full range of movement that pain and stiffness allows. Don't do any heavy exercise. Herbs to relieve inflammation (*Gaultheria*); warm the area (*Camphora, Syzygium, Cajaput*); and repair tissue (*Symphytum*) are added to creams or liniments for daily application. The condition may take six months to resolve so patience and persistence are called for.

Rheumatism (Rheumatoid arthritis) is a disorder of the immune system. Many sufferers are found to have the so-called rheumatic factor, a component of the immune system known as IgM, in their blood. An unknown disturbance causes the immune system to attack the body's own joints and muscles. Hands and feet are most commonly affected but knees, shoulders and spine are also hit. Unlike osteoarthritis, this disease usually affects pairs of joints at the same time. Symptoms usually start slowly from middle age and it tends to run in families. Joint stiffness in the mornings followed by aching, swollen, hot joints, slight fever and tiredness are typical symptoms. Many people escape with mild symptoms that never progress but serious cases end up with swollen, deformed joints and severe pain. Stress and poor diet are known to aggravate the condition and can trigger attacks after periods of freedom from symptoms.

There are many rheumatic diseases apart from rheumatoid arthritis. Polyarteritis nodosa, polymyalgia rheumatica, Reiter's syndrome, psoritic arthritis, and temporal arteritis are examples of related disease processes. Don't assume that aches and pains in the joints or muscles must be either 'old age' or simple rheumatism. Careful investigation is needed before the best treatment can be chosen.

Herbal treatment is possible only after taking a careful and detailed history of the symptoms, noting the patient's general health, emotional state, diet and family history. Treating this disease is as good an example of holistic medicine as can be found. Treatment may need to attend to the immune system, stress and the state of the nervous system, the digestive and eliminative systems, including the kidneys, the adrenal system, and the circulation. The range of herbs that could be considered for an individual patient is enormous. Typical herbs might include anti-inflammatories (*Dioscorea, Menyanthes, Harpogophytum, Salix, Tanacetum*); diuretics, especially those that encourage elimination of uric acid (*Apium, Betula*); adrenal herbs to stimulate the body's own supply of steroids (*Glycyrrhiza, Smilax*); circulation stimulants (*Zanthoxylum, Capsicum, Cola, Tanacetum, Guaiacum*); and liver herbs. Rubs containing anti-inflammatory herbs (*Gaultheria*) and rubifacient, or heating herbs (*Camphor, Capsicum, Rosmarinus, Syzygium*) that draw the blood into the joint, bring relief and promote a calming of the inflammation and thus make the use of the joints easier.

Dietary advice as appropriate, aiming at reducing acid-forming foods, increasing light diuretics such as salads and fruits, and avoiding foods suspected as encouraging the inflammatory response in joints, e.g. tomatoes, potatos, peppers, oranges, and red wines. Dietary supplements that may be considered include zinc, vitamins E and C, and cod liver oil.

Osteoarthritis is often confused with rheumatoid arthritis. This condition is one of wear and tear of joints, usually the weight-bearing joints of the hips and knees. The smooth surfaces of the joints break down and wear away leaving the bones no longer rubbing over a smooth, low friction surface but instead over a rough, irregular surface. Even imagining it is painful.

Single joints are affected usually. Typically there is little early morning pain or stiffness because only after using the worn joints does the pain appear. Pain and aching late in the day, often related to the amount of work joints have done, is characteristic. There is often inflammation after using the joint.

Often rheumatoid arthritis so damages the joints that the joint surfaces are destroyed resulting in osteoarthritis. There is no cure for osteoarthritis. Joint replacement overcomes the problem in severely disabling cases. Treatment focuses on the relief of pain and calming any inflammation. Herbal treatment is similar to the anti-inflammatory herbs used in rheumatism. Adding *Syzygium* or *Acontium* to rubs helps with pain relief. Losing excess weight alone can bring great relief to osteoarthritis of the knee or hip.

Gout is very much alive and well and is not restricted to the portly, wealthy classes who live on smoked salmon, cream sauces and red wine. It is due to the accumulation of uric acid, a normal waste product of nucleoprotein metabolism in the body. Diets rich in nucleoproteins, problems with kidney function, or certain drugs including diuretics, make matters worse. Crystals of uric acid end up in the joint spaces where they cause very painful inflammation. The big toe is the apocryphal site for gout but it can affect any joint.

Treatment involves looking for any obvious cause of high uric acid, cutting purine rich foods (sardines, offals, red meat, pulses, alcohol, caffeine drinks) from the diet and stimulating kidney excretion of uric acid. Herbal treatment is with diuretics that also encourage uric acid elimination (*Apium, Ægopodium,* Asparagus). *Colchicum* has been used for centuries but the side effects are too dangerous.

Backache is common. Most of the time the causes are minor strains and stresses on the joints of the spine and the surrounding muscles. But it can be caused by kidney disease, osteoarthritis, ankalosing spondylosis, or slipped discs. Careful diagnosis is important and when doctors are unsure of the cause it is advisable to see a chiropractor or osteopath, both of whom are specialists in back problems.

Emotional stress is often focused in muscle spasm anywhere from the neck down to the small of the back. Spasms can be painful, and may cause pain also by compressing the spine or causing it to be bent, ending up with pressure on the nerves leaving the spinal cord. One common example is sciatica. There are layers of small muscles up the spine and attached to the ribs. It is remarkable how easily a slight twist of the body, or bending over with everyday weights like a shopping bag, can result in strained or torn muscles along the spine. This is a very common cause of back pain but the patients often disbelieve the diagnosis because they don't remember lifting any heavy weights.

Where muscle strain or spasm from emotional stress are the culprits, herbal treatment is effective rapidly. Rubs with antispasmodics (*Viburnum, Lavandula, Atropa*) and, as necessary, anti-inflammatories (*Gaultheria*), and heating oils (*Cajaput, Rosmarinus, Camphora, Syzygium, Mentha*) are rapidly soothing. Strains also benefit from the use of *Symphytum* which aids the healing of damaged connective tissues. Help spasms due to stress by soaking in a comfortably hot bath to which ten to twenty drops of essential oil of *Lavandula* have been added.

Beware of any of the following symptoms, which may indicate conditions that should be treated by a doctor or herbalist:

- **low backache with fever and nausea**

- **joint pain with fever, rigors in children**

NERVOUS SYSTEM

There is more to the nervous system than the brain and its important functions. In addition are peripheral nerves that leave the spinal cord, taking messages from and delivering instructions to muscles and organs. These nerves, together with the processing centre or brain, make up most of the voluntary nervous system, allowing us to walk, lift and manipulate objects and sense touch, heat and pain, etc.

There is also an involuntary or autonomic nervous system which keeps important bodily functions and their regulation running smoothly without us having to think about them. It is like being on autopilot. This is made up of two distinct parts, the sympathetic and the parasympathetic. The sympathetic or 'flight and fight' nerves also leave the spinal cord and are interconnected through junctions or ganglia laid in a chain on either side of the spine. These nerves contact organs like the heart, intestines and blood vessels. Under stress they act to increase heartbeat, shift blood into muscles ready for action, constrict the pupils, and increase sweating of the palms and soles of the feet to increase friction and make fighting or getting away easier. The parasympathetic part has an opposite calming effect on the body. Its actions include slowing the activity of the heart, stimulating release of digestive juices, allowing the bladder to be emptied, and sexual arousal to occur. Most of this system is supplied by one nerve starting in the base of the brain and travelling down the middle of the body, where it connects with the heart and intestines. Small parts of four other nerves arising from the brain are also parasympathetics and spread over the head where they control activities like the iris of the eye and salivary glands. Some smaller nerves leaving the very bottom of the spinal cord control the bladder and anus.

A related part of the autonomic nervous system is a specialized area of the brain, the hypothalamus. This is like the computer control panel keeping the main services (air-conditioning, room temperature, waste disposal) of a modern factory or office block running smoothly. The hypothalamus regulates our blood pressure, the amount of water lost in urine, body temperature, appetite. These are controlled by nerve signals fed to the sympathetic nerves, but the hypothalamus also stimulates the pituitary (lying just beneath the hypothalamus in the centre of the brain) which releases six important hormones into the blood. The hormones turn on or off the supply of other hormones that are released from glands like the thyroid, adrenals, and ovaries. Because hormones change what the body does, and how, they are similar to nerves in their effects on controlling the body.

The nervous system is an extraordinary means of controlling the human body but this control is easily disrupted by stress which is either too prolonged or too severe. There are many sources and degrees of stress. It can be due to excess physical activity, serious illness, shift work, the emotional stresses of life. Many common illnesses are caused directly by disordered behaviour of the nervous system. These are called psychosomatic or functional illnesses. Typical examples are nervous indigestion, irritable bowel syndrome, skin rashes, painful periods, insomnia, and even an overactive thyroid gland.

Herbal medicine is well designed both to ease the effects of stress on the body and strengthen and to repair the nervous system. In the medicinal plant cupboard are herbs that can have a wide range of specific actions on the nervous system. There are herbs that can relax, tranquillize, enhance mood (thymoleptics), reverse depression (antidepressants), calm anxiety (anxiolytics), stimulate, encourage sleep (hypnotic), relieve pain (anodynes), relieve spasm, sedate, and anaesthetize. With this armoury many common problems involving the nervous system can be helped.

Anxiety and depression are often closely related. Anxiety is an extreme form of normal reactions of alertness or awareness. First signs of anxiety may be excessive worry over ordinary daily events, feelings of doom and disaster dominating thought. Sufferers tend to be restless, have panics over minor problems and sleep poorly. They are unable to concentrate and this tends to increase their failure to manage their situation. Depression may follow.

Physical symptoms are often noticed first as many people either deny their anxiety or don't realize it is the cause of their discomfort. Headaches, back or neck pain, palpitations, indigestion, bloating, diarrhoea, dizziness, insomnia, and fatigue are commonly presented to herbalists for treatment. Often the underlying cause is anxiety.

Everyone is depressed or 'down' after events like the death of a pet or losing a job. These coping crises are understandable and usually shortlived. A person is usually described as clinically depressed when their depression is deeper and more prolonged than usual. Depressed people usually lose interest in themselves and others, they no longer smile but look sad and gloomy all the time. They have little to say, and tend to see the blackest side of their and every other situation. Many symptoms are common with anxiety, but, in depression, despair and hopelessness are more severe and the person may even talk of suicide.

With both anxiety and depression, the causes are most often to do with circumstances surrounding people. Careful talking with the sufferer can identify possible causes and help find resolutions. Counselling may be helpful, especially where there are no family or friends the sufferer can talk to with trust and confidence. Some causes are due to chemical problems in the working of the brain, and psychiatric help may be needed.

Herbalists can help with focusing attention on locating the causes of anxiety and depression. Herbs that can help while the problems are being tackled include anxiolytics (*Scutellaria*) to calm feelings of panic; relaxants (*Melissa, Valeriana, Verbena*); antidepressants (*Hypericum, Damiana*); hypnotics to help with sleeping (*Passiflora*); thymoleptics to lift mood (*Borago*). Where anxiety is the dominant feature and there is no depression, sedating herbs can be useful to slow down any overreactions (*Piscidia, Lactuca, Humulus*).

Insomnia is deceptively simple. Herbalists are confronted with patients complaining they cannot sleep and requesting a 'sleeping draught'. There is frustration when the herbalist explains that they cannot know what herbs will help until they learn *why* there is insomnia. There are as many reasons for sleeping badly as there are patterns on pyjamas.

Anxiety is one of the most common causes and is suggested by waking one or more times during the night. To wake at the same hour each night is typical. But ulcers, indigestion, shift work which disturbs the body clock, caffeine drinks before bed, back problems, and some drugs can all disturb sleep. Elderly people, who need only four to six hours sleep a night, may complain of insomnia because they think they should be having at least eight hours.

Herbalists approach the problem through its causes. Anxiety or depression would be tackled. High caffeine and alcoholic drinks should be avoided before bed. Thought should be given to either relaxing activity like reading or physical activity to promote tiredness; calming baths with essential oil of lavender before bed; checking the comfort of the mattress and room temperature or ventilation; and banishing snoring partners or pets; all are worthy of consideration. In their place herbs, to promote sleep (*Passiflora*); to sedate (*Lactuca, Piscidia, Eschscholzia, Humulus*); to relax (*Valeriana*); to relieve anxiety (*Scutellaria*); could be combined according to each person's needs.

Headaches and migraines are among the most uncomfortable of pains. Headaches can be aching or throbbing and can affect different parts of the head, even different sides of the head. The pain can move about and change in character. The causes are many, usually not serious, but any headache that doesn't respond to simple self-treatment after forty-eight hours should be investigated. Inflammation or constriction of blood vessels in the scalp or of those supplying the sensitive meninges membrane surrounding the brain are the most common triggers. Digestive problems, stress, noise, breathing too little oxygen or noxious vapours, eye strain, and bad posture or problems in the neck vertebrae can precipitate headaches. Other diseases, including high blood pressure, diabetes, infections causing fever, sinusitis, temporal arteritis, brain tumours, and brain haemorrhages can also cause headaches so they should never be dismissed as mere unpleasant inconveniences.

Migraines are headaches associated with warning signs (prodromes) like blurred vision and flashing lights in the eyes. They are usually severe, throbbing headaches accompanied by nausea and vomiting, intolerance of bright lights, and sometimes temporary paralysis in the arms. Stress is known to trigger migraines, often at weekends after the stress of the workplace has been left behind. Foods (chocolate, caffeine, cheeses, food additives) and the changing concentrations of female hormones have been shown to trigger attacks. Cluster headaches are migraine-type headaches that occur in groups, even as often as daily, over periods of days or weeks with long gaps between the clusters.

Abdominal migraine is an unrelated condition where young children complain of stomach pains and discomfort. No evidence of the symptoms is found. The cause is usually stress.

Headaches are divided roughly into throbbing or aching, 'hot' or 'cold', migrainous, and other types. 'Hot' headaches feel better with a cold pack whereas 'cold' headaches are relieved with a hot pack on the head. The former suggests the presence of dilated blood vessels, which are contracted by the cold pack, returning the blood flow to normal and reducing the throbbing. The 'cold' type reflect spasm in the arteries where the heat encourages dilation to restore normal flow.

Herbal treatment depends on knowing the type of headache as much as any identifiable causes. Stress headaches benefit from relieving the body's response to stress and avoiding or removing stress where possible. Relaxant herbs (*Valeriana, Verbena, Melissa*) are indicated, especially *Stachys betonica,* which is specific for headaches. Rubbing essential oil of lavender into the back of the neck muscles relieves spasm headaches. 'Cold' types, which include many migraines, call for vasodilatory remedies like feverfew (*Tanacetum*), *Tilia,* and *Ginkgo.* 'Hot' headaches are commonly stress and tension 'throbbers' and benefit from relaxant herbs plus digestive and liver herbs, notably the bitters. Occasionally herbs to constrict the blood vessels are useful (*Sarothamnus*) but care is necessary. Many headaches begin with constriction but become dilatory. Generally calming herbs to relax the person and antispasmodics to calm tension in the viscera and muscles of the neck and head are helpful. One recommendable example is the taking of a warm bath to which 10-15 drops of essential oil of lavender have been added.

ME or myalgic encephalomyelitis remains a conundrum. Diagnostic criteria are wide and could be explained by many other conditions. The causes are uncertain, the number of sufferers difficult to identify or agree upon. However, what was dismissed as purely psychosomatic only a few years ago, is accepted, despite the difficulties in diagnosis or explanation, as a distinct health problem.

Patients show common symptoms of nervous system dysfunction. Muscles ache after exercise, they have poor concentration, short-term memory loss, clumsiness, chronic tiredness, and disturbance of the autonomic nervous system. Many are depressed, though it is difficult to unravel the effect of having the ME symptoms as a cause of depression.

Herbal treatment focuses on the specific history and symptoms of each ME patient, but there are general guidelines. The viral background in most sufferers suggests immune system stimulation (*Echinacea, Astralagus*), general adaptogen treatment to lift the overall metabolic performance (*Elutherococcus*) and circulatory stimulants to improve blood flow in the brain (*Ginkgo*). Specific symptoms like stomach pain, palpitations, and insomnia can be helped as they arise in each patient.

Beware of any of the following symptoms, which may indicate conditions that should be treated by a doctor or herbalist:

- headaches that occur every morning on waking

- regular headaches accompanied by nausea or vomiting

- any fall or blow to the head that may have resulted in being knocked out, even briefly, and which was followed by nausea or loss of memory

---

URINARY DISEASES

The two kidneys are precisely designed selective filtration devices. They filter blood under pressure, holding back the blood cells but channelling the filtrate down fine tubules which reabsorb most of the water and solutes back into the body. The discarded liquid is the urine, in which are soluble waste chemicals, together with excess salts and water. But the kidney is not a mere drain. It is cleverly designed to regulate the composition of the blood and body fluids so that waste water and other chemicals are discarded only when it is necessary to maintain balance in the body. In a sense the kidneys and their urine represent a balancing act between what is taken through the mouth and what the body needs to keep or dispose of.

There are other important organs of balance, especially the skin, the lungs, and the bowels, which also eliminate waste. But the kidney is the most impressive in fine tuning and precision. A healthy pair of kidneys is essential for good health. As part of the herbalist's concern for bodily function, the kidneys need to be efficient. Each one of the pair contains over a million special filters with their sensitive tubules. Every hour, about forty litres of blood are squeezed into each kidney's filters and all but about 30ml are reabsorbed into the blood. All the blood in the body passes through the kidneys around 15-18 times a day. Urine is passed only when the amount of water drunk daily meets the body's needs and leaves a surplus to pass via the kidneys. This is why we pass less urine in hot weather compared to cold winter days when we sweat much less.

Urinary tract infections cover serious infections like glomeronephritis and pyelonephritis, which are infections within the kidney, as well as infections in the tubules carrying the urine from the kidneys to the bladder and from the bladder in the single urethra to the outside. It is not always easy to distinguish exactly where the infection is from the symptoms alone. In adults there may be pain in the loin and tenderness over the pubic area and loin, with fever and even rigors. Painful and frequent urination are typical. Pus may make the urine cloudy to the naked eye and blood may be visible. In infants there may be none of these symptoms, only malaise and fever with that typical 'white as a sheet' appearance and restlessness. Urine tests looking for bacteria, blood, and protein in the urine are routine diagnostic tests but even positive findings do not always make for a clear diagnosis.

Infections can arise from transfer of bacteria like *E. coli* from the bowel to the opening of the urethra, from where it travels up the urinary tubules. Sexual intercourse and pregnancy are common causes that are easily overlooked. But infections can also arise from the blood being pumped into the kidneys. The bacteria then travel down the tubes. Diabetics are particularly prone because they have excess sugar, a favourite food of bacteria, in their urine.

Simple lower urinary tract infection is best illustrated by cystitis. Men as well as women can suffer but women, having the shorter path from the urethral opening to the bladder, are affected more often. Well recognized symptoms are excruciating pain on passing urine, especially on finishing. The misery is compounded by a tendency to pass urine more often than usual. Sufferers usually have repeated attacks.

Herbal treatment is fourfold. Stimulating the immune system can help stop recurrent attacks. The immediate pain can be eased with a mixture of herbs that disinfect the tubules (*Barosma, Arctostaphylos, Vaccinum*); that soothe the inflamed tubule walls (*Agropyron, Zea, Althaea*); and that stop bleeding and heal inflammation (*Equisetum*). These should be taken as a tea and drunk regularly from the first twinge.

Kidney stones and gravel cause terrible pain known as renal colic. Sufferers recognize it as one of the most severe pains imaginable and sometimes can trace moving stones as the pain travels diagonally from the loin to the pubic area. Sometimes the stones or fine gravel are passed out in the urine. This may cause bleeding and, to add insult to injury, increases the chances of a following infection.

The best approach is preventive. Both acid and alkaline urines can deposit stones. The solution is to ensure sufficient fluid is drunk to produce a volume of dilute urine daily. The pain of urinary colic is treated effectively by herbalists with strong painkillers (*Hyoscyamus*) that are not available to the public and should never be used by the untrained.

Bedwetting is usually due to anxiety or neuroses, whether in children or adults. Herbalists assess the nature and causes in each case and can help identify successful treatments. Herbs that are useful include relaxants (*Valerian*); antispasmodics (*Viburnum*, *Atropa*); and antidepressants (*Hypericum*), often mixed with urinary astringents (*Equisetum*) that are toning of the urinary bladder and the sphincters (muscles that allow release of urine).

REPRODUCTIVE SYSTEM PROBLEMS

Herbs are particularly suited to many of the functional hiccups of both the male and female reproductive systems. Apart from the machinery of the genitals, the system relies for most efficient functioning on delicate balances of a string of hormones supplied from different glands around the body. Like most animals, the design of the human reproductive process is clumsy and it often requires both nurture and support to work smoothly. Herbs offer a rich source of hormonal mimic ingredients that help with hormone-related problems.

Menstrual problems include pain, lack of or infrequent periods, and excessive flow. Pain can be of the spasmodic type that peaks as the period begins and lasts for only a few hours. This is often relieved after the first vaginal birth, but not by Caesarean deliveries. The congestive type of pain may start several days before or continue one or more days into the period. These have different causes and need careful diagnosis before appropriate treatment can be designed. Endometriosis, pelvic congestion and even a displaced uterus could be responsible. Problems with the length, regularity or frequency of the cycle can be related to a string of problems. Certainly a lack of periods may be physiological due to youth or old age or, surprisingly often, it is due to an unrecognized pregnancy. Heavy dieting and anorexia can lead the body to make the wise decision to stop periods because of malnutrition. Hormonal disturbances are common in emotional stress and even time-clock changes due to international travel. Anxiety can delay periods by up to two weeks.

Constant or prolonged bleeding, even with varying amounts and character of flow, suggests problems. Many women bleed slightly or 'show' at ovulation. This is not a cause for concern. Prolonged bleeding may indicate fibroids or even uterine cancer.

Heavy menstrual blood loss is both a sign of abnormality and a potential cause of anaemia. Endometriosis and fibroids are suggested and it should always be investigated.

Herbalists use antispasmodics (*Viburnum opulus, Viburnum prunifolium, Caulophyllum, Cimicifuga*), and pain relievers (*Anemone*) backed with herbs aimed at the causes of the pelvic congestion where necessary (*Zanthoxylum, Calendula, Matricaria, Chamaelirium*). For endometriosis, fibroids, and excessive bleeding *Mitchella, Capsella, Trillium* and *Vinca* could be chosen.

Irregular periods may be treated with *Chamaelirium, Vitex, Alchemilla, Angelica sinensis*. Lack of periods (amenorrhoea) used to be treated with herbs that act as emmenagogues. These herbs stimulate the uterine muscle and are technically abortifacient so should always be used with great caution.

Premenstrual tension (PMT) produces variable symptoms that include mood swings, clumsiness, sugar and chocolate cravings, water retention, bloating, swollen and painful breasts. The cause is unclear but it is thought that a combination of altered release of pituitary hormones that control the initiation of follicle growth in the ovaries, progesterone release during the menstrual cycle, and the possible hypersecretion of oestrogen in the second half of the cycle may be involved. In short there may be a shortage of progesterone or a relative excess of oestrogen behind the symptoms.

Herbalists use *Vitex*, which has been shown to alter the balance of the LH (luteinizing hormone) and FSH (follicle stimulating hormone) hormones released from the pituitary, with the result of increasing progesterone in relation to oestrogen. The treatment takes up to three cycles to be fully effective and when successful appears to have 'reset' the pituitary and the medication can be stopped. Taking evening primrose oil during the last half of the cycle and avoiding both coffee and chocolate can have dramatic benefits. Other herbs can be used to reduce the water retention (*Taraxacum, Parietaria*); calm the mood swings and headaches (*Stachys, Vervain, Matricaria*); and relieve the constipation often found before periods (*Taraxacum, Rumex*).

Menopause struggles afflict some women but bypass others totally. With the end of the active ovaries comes a sudden drop in the regular production of copious supplies of the hormone oestrogen. This is the calming, softening, nurturing hormone of the menstrual cycle. As it is withdrawn it is as though the body misses the calming influence and it becomes uncontrollably 'heated'. The unpleasant symptoms of flushing, night sweats, weight gain, irritability and depression increase steadily as the regularity of periods breaks up and eventually stops. Both the severity of symptoms and their duration vary among women. Eventually the body readjusts to the new low level of oestrogen and life settles down to the mellow autumnal years, which for many women are sheer delight without the monthly burden of periods.

Hormone replacement therapy is not recommended simply to avoid the symptoms of entering menopause. It has unpleasant side effects and only delays the menopause. When the HRT is stopped eventually, the body still has to enter menopause. HRT is best kept for strict medical needs, such as immediately after a total hysterectomy without complications of cancer.

Herbalists help with plants that calm the body's overreaction to lowered oestrogen (*Alchemilla, Leonurus, Artemesia vulgaris, Chamaelirium*). Night sweats can be helped with *Atropa*, but this herb should be tried only on a prescription from a herbalist. After the menopause the vagina reduces in both size and elasticity. Arousal secretions dry up but sexual desire doesn't. Using a light marigold (*Calendula*) cream before having sex removes the dryness and helps heal any minor abrasions to the delicate internal wall.

Pelvic inflammations cover several conditions, the most important of which are salpingitis (inflamed fallopian tubes) and uterine infections. The cause can be from venereal infections like gonorrhoea or *Chlamydia*, from IUD's, miscarriages, abortions, or from infections already within the abdomen. There is usually a dark discharge with pain low in the pelvis, on one or both sides, and fever. The other tell-tale symptom to raise the alarm is pain on sexual intercourse or on touching the cervix.

Infections in the 'tubes' are not common but can be serious as they can cause infertility or even spread the infection to the abdomen resulting in peritonitis. The symptoms can be confused with other conditions (endometriosis, ectopic pregnancy, and appendicitis). As with most problems in the female pelvis, the only safe diagnosis is via a gynaecologist who may well perform a laparoscopy. This is the only way to diagnose many conditions and involves inserting a small flexible telescope through a tiny slit in the abdomen so the action can be seen. This allows for earlier and more accurate diagnosis.

Treatment of the acute condition may require antibiotics. Plenty of bedrest is usually advised. Herbalists are more suitable to help with the chronic forms of pelvic inflammation resulting from problems of congestion or tissue damage after acute infections. Here they use toning herbs (*Chamaelirium, Hydrastis, Seneico aureus*); circulatory herbs for the pelvis (*Crateagus, Senecio, Thuja, Calendula*); possibly with anti-infectives where there is a suspected chronic low-grade infection (*Echinacea, Baptisia*). The pain could be relieved with *Pulsatilla* and *Viburnum*.

Vaginitis and cervicitis take many forms but are more irritating than serious. Often a bacterial infection is the cause but tampons and other foreign bodies or inserted chemicals (douches, lubricants, pessaries) are equally likely causes. The vaginal tissues are well armed with natural defences against bacterial attacks and a breach usually suggests a weakened immune system. Sufferers often have a history of infections elsewhere, including cystitis and thrush as well.

After menopause vaginal secretions cease and the walls of the vagina are more susceptible to abrasion, which leads to inflammation. Cervicitis is very common after childbirth and may exist for years before being detected. Symptoms include irritation in the vagina and vulva, discharges that change in character with different bacterial infections.

If an infection is suspected go first to a doctor. Herbalists can treat with local anti-inflammatories (*Calendula, Matricaria*); and toning herbs (*Lamium, Trillium*); backed by internal herbs against infection (*Echinacea, Allium, Baptisia*); and to tone the area (*Chamaelirium, Myrica, Senecio*). Where the person is generally run down *Elutherococcus* could be used to help strengthen the body's systems, including the immune system.

Thrush is very common and women seem to put up with recurrent attacks as though there were no choice. The fungal cause, *Candida albicans*, lives naturally within all of us but becomes a nuisance only when there is uncontrolled growth. This usually occurs when there has been a disturbance of the immune system, often following a period of illness or stress, or because of poor eating habits. There is a red rash around and often in the vagina, severe itching and discomfort, and a thick curdling white discharge. It is not uncommon to find thrush infections in the mouth or intestines at the same time.

Herbalists look for the reasons why the immune system is oppressed and set about righting those where possible. Specific treatment for thrush involves internal medicines to lift the immune system (*Echinacea, Elutherococcus*) and general metabolic functioning. Herb choices might include nervines (*Verbena, Hypericum*), toning herbs (*Hydrastis*) and bitters for the liver (*Gentiana, Berberis, Artemesia*). Creams and pessaries for the vagina can tackle the fungus head on (*Calendula, Lamium, Melaleuca*).

Threatened miscarriage Herbalists are reluctant to treat pregnant women with anything that is not essential. Help with threatened miscarriage is one exception. The first three months of pregnancy are the most hazardous, as many women find to their cost with repeated miscarriages. Although miscarriages may happen earlier and are more often than realized nature's way of stopping a damaged foetus developing, they also occur because of functional problems in the nurturing womb. Herbalists can reduce the chances of these 'misbehaving womb' miscarriages. Herbs that specifically tone and calm the uterine tissues are particularly useful (*Chamaelirium, Cimicifuga, Viburnum*).

Herbs to avoid in pregnancy:

Berberis, Gossypium, Ruta, Thuja, Salvia, Juniperus, Artemesia, Petroselinum, Apium, Hydrastis, Tanacetum.

Childbirth Midwives regularly either prescribe raspberry leaf tea remedies before birth or encourage their charges to bring their own supplies into hospital or the home for labour. The leaves of both raspberry (*Rubus idaeus*) and wild blackberry have a calming antispasmodic effect on the pregnant uterus helping it relax and not go into painful spasms during the rhythmic contractions of labour. The tea is drunk regularly during the last six weeks of the pregnancy and during labour. Other herbs that help in easing labour and delivery are *Caulophyllum* and *Cimicifuga*.

Sore nipples are a hazard of breast feeding. The physical gnawing of little gums, the effect of constant moisture, and the rubbing of inflamed nipples against underwear invites trouble. Herbalists use a simple and extremely soothing cream of *Calendula* and *Matricaria* to protect from moisture, heal inflammation and any cracks.

Beware of any of the following symptoms, which may indicate conditions that should be treated by a doctor or herbalist:

- at the first signs or fears of a miscarriage report to the midwife or doctor

- painless vaginal bleeding that continues outside expected periods or after menopause

- any new breast lump or swelling, especially if it changes in size

BABIES AND CHILDREN

When adults are ill they tend to play it down, even when they need medical attention. Ill babies and children produce a different reaction in adults. Parents and carers are more likely to overreact to the slightest deviation from the normal.

Babies take time to develop efficient organs and their immune system. In the first months and years, they are more delicate and react to slight disturbances in their diet or to minor infections. Stomach and bowel disturbances are common and body temperature bobs up and down more easily and more often than in older children and adults. Towards the teens, bodies are growing rapidly and are put through stress and strains as play gets more active. Early school years expose children to large numbers of other children leading to greater sharing of infectious diseases. The immune system is still creating and storing its identification records on threatening bacteria and viruses, and is thus still weaker than it becomes after puberty and into adulthood. Young children collect 'childhood diseases' like chicken pox, measles and mumps as their teenage siblings collect pop idols and fashionable clothing.

Herbal medicine is particularly suited to the treatment of babies and children. Their healthy bodies may be strong but not robust enough for the heavy-handed effects of many pharmaceutical drugs. Herbs are both gentle on the body and effective for the majority of common illnesses affecting babies and children. Most illnesses are minor and can be treated effectively and safely at home with herbs. Where there is any doubt or uncertainty about a diagnosis or the rate of healing, do not hesitate. Go to the doctor or herbalist to get a diagnosis. Once you know what is happening and that it is a normal path for a particular condition, you will find generally that you can still treat with herbs but will have much greater confidence. If it is something that needs other treatment, you will be advised and will be thankful for your prudent checking.

Children have less reserve and control than adults and thus react to stress more directly, if not always more vocally. Stress can come from all manner of sources and has direct effects on the emotional and physical health of children. Parents may overlook the possibility of stress at home when looking at their child's health. Herbalists are trained to include both the environmental and emotional elements of every patient's health and are especially aware of the possibility of stress in children. This is important because most common childhood illnesses involve emotional stress sometimes, if not all the time. Conditions in which stress has a causal role include bedwetting, sleeplessness, repeated infections of throat etc., headaches, stomach upsets, recurrent 'fevers', loss of appetite, general but non-specific pains.

With children, even more than with adults, the essence of the herbal approach is in promoting health rather than treating disease. Freedom from avoidable stresses and traumas, plenty of mental and physical stimulation, peaceful rest with sufficient sleep, together with healthy food and a relaxing environment in which to eat it are the essentials of healthy development.

Fever Average temperature is 36.8°C (98.4°F) but may be a few parts of a degree above or below. Children's temperatures fluctuate more than adults. It is common for the temperature to rise to 38°C (100.4°F) or even 38.5°C (101.3°F) without there being any cause for alarm. On the other hand children can be ill without there being any rise in temperature, so observe their behaviour carefully. The child may not even appear restless or uncomfortable with a slight fever. When the temperature rises to 39.5-40°C (103.1-104°F), the fever is too high. The child should be bathed in tepid water to bring the temperature down slightly.

Slight fever is a natural response to infection and should not be lowered habitually with aspirin or paracetamol. When the fever begins, the body's thermostat is still set below the rising temperature and so the body sweats in an attempt to cool it. Once the 'top of the fever' has been reached, the thermostat slowly adjusts and then it 'resets' to the higher temperature. When the body's temperature begins to fall, the new higher setting suggests to the brain that the falling temperature is abnormally low and the body begins to shiver in an attempt to keep the temperature up. This is a useful sign because it means that when there is shivering in a fever, the crisis is past and the body is returning to normal.

Herbal treatment recognizes the important function of slight fever and encourages it. Whenever a child has fever, it is important to find out what has caused it. There are usually other symptoms or signs: catarrh and red throat in colds and flu; swollen tonsils and glands in tonsillitis; cough in bronchitis; diarrhoea possibly with vomiting in digestive upsets etc. These conditions need appropriate treatment. For the fever, herbalists might use *Sambucus, Tilia, Nepeta*, or *Achillea* to help control the fever. *Sambucus* (elder) berries are better than the flowers for children because they have another useful action. They are slightly laxative (aperient) which helps reverse the constipation that usually accompanies cold or flu fevers in children.

Colds and sore throats have nothing to do with getting wet in the rain or running about without a shirt. They are due to infections by viruses and bacteria. But they are caused by the body's defences being weakened, which allows the bacteria or viruses to enter the tissues. The symptoms are merely the body's reaction to a rampaging infectious agent. Remember we are covered in bacteria and are constantly breathing in air laden with virus-rich droplets, fungal spores and bacteria, but only rarely do we get infected. The healthy body has a remarkably effective protective mechanism.

A cold starts with a sore throat, but young children may not complain. Soon enough the well-known dripping nose is followed by a thicker yellow-green discharge and cough. The infection may start with a virus but bacteria soon take hold and the condition may get worse. The tonsils, adenoids, and sinuses may be involved and the infection often travels down into the throat and lungs. Especially in young children, the narrow tubes connecting the back of the throat to the middle ear, the eustachian tubes, are easily infected from coughing, which forces catarrh up the tubes and the infection can travel to the middle ear. This can cause earache and, if serious infection follows, glue ear may result.

Herbalists see frequent sore throats and colds as signs of a weakened immune system. Diet, a weakened metabolism, physical or emotional exhaustion, and even regular doses of antibiotics can weaken the immune system. Treatment might include dietary advice and help with sleep or emotional problems where they are leading to exhaustion. Herbal remedies could include bitters to promote the digestive system; herbs to stimulate the immune system (*Echinacea*); anti-infective herbs where the infection is rampant (*Baptisia, Allium, Thymus*); anticatarrhals to tone and dry up the mucous membranes of the nose, Eustachian tubes and the upper respiratory tract generally (*Glechoma, Plantago, Sambucus, Hydrastis*); and, if relevant, anti-infectives and expectorants for the throat and lungs (*Hyssopus, Inula, Allium, Elecampane, Urginea*). Sore throats respond well to astringent herbs taken as a gargle (*Salvia, Quercus, Myrrh*). Where there are swollen tonsils or adenoids, and the glands under the jaw and in the sides of the neck and head are up, herbs to help include *Calendula, Phytolacca, Echinacea, Populus*.

Glue ear and middle-ear infections are more common in young children and babies because their eustachian tubes are shorter and infections can more easily reach the chamber of the middle ear than in older children or adults. There is the added complication that young immune systems are not very resistant to the assaults of life.

Glue ear is what it sounds like. The infection in the middle ear causes the same thick mucus and pus that is found in infections of the nose, sinuses or throat. But, as with sinus infections, it is not easy for the muck to drain away. The worse the infection, and the longer it goes on untreated, the thicker and more copious the mucus in the ear. This thick mucus builds up pressure in what is normally an air-filled cavity and does two things. First, it presses on the walls and eardrum causing pain and eventually it may burst through the drum causing a thick and copious discharge from the ear. Second, it gums up or 'glues' the three tiny bones in the middle ear that carry sound signals from the drum to the auditory nerve. The result is temporary deafness and if the eardrum is repeatedly ruptured and the ear constantly 'glued' up, there can be permanent deafness.

Herbalists look for the early evidence of either repeated infections or catarrhal states in children. Prevention beats cure and glue ear can be prevented. Catarrhal states may be due to diet, dust, allergies (allergic rhinitis), or, in young children, chronic mild infection of the upper respiratory tract. These are treated appropriately. Although there may be earache warning of a catarrhal blockage in the ear, this is not always evident, especially in young babies who suffer pain stoically. Sometimes they rub the affected ear. There may be a fever with the infection but this too is not always present.

When glue ear is presented, careful decisions are needed. If there is already a copious discharge, rupture of the drum has already occurred. This cannot be checked immediately because the discharge usually fills the ear canal and the drum cannot be seen with the viewing instrument. If the discharge has been present for several days, or the child is seen before rupture of the drum and it appears very red and bulging, it is worth considering antibiotics. Ear infections can be difficult to budge and the risks of long-term damage make middle ear infections legitimate candidates for antibiotics. However, if the infection is in its early stages or the patient appears between regular attacks, then herbal treatment can be both appropriate and very effective.

Herbal treatment aims to dry the catarrh, stop the infection, boost the immune system to stop further attacks, and reduce any catarrhal encouragement in the child's diet or environment. Useful herbs include *Echinacea, Glechoma, Plantago, Eucalyptus,* and *Sambucus.* So long as the eardrum has not ruptured, ear drops of infused oils (*Hypericum, Verbascum*) with a few drops of essential oil of *Eucalyptus* ease earache and calm the inflamed drum. If the drum is ruptured, do not use any ear drops.

Colic affects babies more than older children or adults, but is still overstated, over-treated, and over soon enough. Babies swallow air with their food and their tendency to lie about on their backs with their legs waving in the air encourages the passing of wind from their mouth and rectum. This is natural. Crying after food is more likely to be due to either eating too much, indigestion because of the food (e.g. from bananas, cow's milk, apple, coarse cereal), or swallowing air.

The best herbal treatment is with carminatives. These are usually seeds rich in aromatic oils (anise, caraway, fennel) or other plant parts also rich in these oils (*Matricaria, Melissa*). The action is to stimulate the whole digestive process as well as toning the walls of the intestine, reducing the tendency to spasm which certainly may cause both pain and trapping of wind. Carminatives are best taken as infusions and can be given to babies after feeding instead of milk.

Diarrhoea and vomiting can occur together but as often are separate incidents. They can have common causes. Diarrhoea is not just a loose stool but a watery stool. In many western countries most people are constipated, passing too large and too firm stools normally. For them, any softening is seen as abnormal, but this should not be confused with being unhealthy. It is common sense that a healthy stool is soft enough to pass easily. Such stools look like curling ribbons once in the lavatory pan and were they passed onto the ground they would resemble a firm cow-pat. That is *not diarrhoea* but a sign of a healthy bowel.

Diarrhoea is a symptom not a disease. Many simple disturbances may be behind the bowel disturbance. Shock or emotional upset, mild fevers, the 'wrong' foods or infections of the stomach and intestine could be responsible. Gastroenteritis or mild food poisoning are common causes in children. Symptoms may be sudden and there may be some pain, but this diarrhoea generally lasts only one or two days and is not serious. Children who eat, drink and behave normally with their diarrhoea are no cause for concern. Only if there is vomiting and fever with the diarrhoea should there be cause for concern. This may be due to food poisoning and could lead to dehydration if it continues more than two or three days.

Treatment is conservative, which means plenty of fluids and only low-fat, simple foods when there is appetite. If there is vomiting as well, collect a sample of the diarrhoea and report to the doctor who can arrange for a laboratory test to see if particular bugs are the cause.

Herbalists approach diarrhoea with relaxants where indicated; with mild astringents (*Agrimonia, Avens, Potentilla*) to calm the lining of the intestine; with antimicrobials (*Allium*); or anti-inflammatories (*Filipendula, Matricaria, Dioscorea*).

Vomiting may be due to simple causes like car or motion sickness, over-eating, too rich a diet, emotions, or excessive physical activity. Infections from colds to gastroenteritis can also cause vomiting. If there is uncontrollable projectile vomiting there may be a serious condition called pyloric stenosis where there is a blockage to the food leaving the stomach. It can also be caused by medical drugs irritating the stomach lining or by inflammation of the liver or gall bladder. Generally, vomiting, like diarrhoea, is not serious. If it persists for more than forty-eight hours, report to a herbalist or doctor.

Like diarrhoea, vomiting is best watched and observed for the first twenty-four hours with the patient calm and warm in bed. Avoid any rich food, but encourage drinking water or lightly sweetened herbal infusions of calming herbs (*Melissa*), carminatives (*Mentha, Foeniculum*), or anti-emetics (*Ballota*).

Teething comes to many babies as the first example of the inbuilt pain of living lurking amongst the pleasures. Few babies escape the pain. Crying and restless nights are the first signs of teething. During the waking hours, there is restlessness, possible slight fever and much putting of fingers into the mouth in desperation.

Herbs can ease the pain (*Matricaria, Melissa*), soothe the inflammation around the erupting teeth (*Filipendula, Matricaria*), and help relax and calm the agitated nervous system (*Tilia*). These are very safe herbs, even for babies. Give only as weak infusions. Clove oil (*Syzygium*) is used as a local anaesthetic, rubbing a drop onto the painful gums. This is not advised for babies, but could be used when the molars appear at about three years of age.

Nappy rash frightens parents because they imagine how uncomfortable they would feel with such a red rash around the groin. It is not the nappy that causes the rash, but the contact of a wet nappy against the skin. Matters are made worse by the acidity of the urine passed and the formation of ammonia in urine stored in a wet and soiled nappy. Modern disposables can make matters worse. They are lined with plastic, which waterproofs the outside of the nappy and allows parents to leave the wet nappy in place for longer than with the old, and less easily ignored, towelling nappies.

Sometimes the nappy rash may be due to thrush, which produces a similar appearance but may also be found elsewhere on the body, especially in the mouth.

Herbalists encourage more sympathetic nappy routines as the best preventive approach. Creams and ointments based on

Calendula are specific. The creams are best made slightly oily as this provides more of a surface barrier, keeping the urine off the skin. The *Calendula* is both anti-inflammatory, soothing the rash, and antifungal, attacking the organism causing any thrush.

Cradle cap is one form of a harmless condition called seborrhoeic dermatitis, which basically means inflammation of areas of oily skin. The scalp, nose folds, and backs of the ears tend to produce more oil than other areas. Some babies are oilier than others, which is why not all babies get cradle cap, nor do babies who suffer its indignity suffer all the time.

The scalp is most commonly affected and thick brownish scales are produced. These come away on washing the hair but may reappear.

Herbalists use an infusion of *Calendula* to which one part of distilled witch-hazel water (*Hamamelis*) is added. If the condition persists or spreads, *Calendula* cream is best. It softens the flakes, making them easier to remove and also soothes the inflammation.

Eczema is an outward sign of internal disorder (See Skin, hair and nails). It covers a multitude of skin conditions that are best described as dermatitis, that is 'inflamed skin'. The rash can be dry or weepy, but both forms are itchy and produce a fine scale. Childhood is when most people suffer eczema, if ever. Whatever the immediate cause, most children leave their eczema behind them by the age of ten or so. Some develop what is called atopy, and have atopic eczema. Atopy is simply the inbuilt tendency to overreact to allergens but the explanation is less simple. No-one yet understands why. The triad of eczema, asthma and hay fever are all usually suffered by atopic children. Atopic eczema is less easy to prevent or treat than other forms.

Eczema may be caused by contact with an irritant or allergen (exogenous) but the condition is still due to an abnormal response from the body's immune system. Metals, soap powders, rubber, lanolin, clothing dyes, synthetic fabric, and chlorine are common triggers.

With children the most common factors found in the eczema

picture are 'hot' constitutions, early weaning onto cow's milk formulas, foods like oranges, eggs, tomatoes, and food dyes. Often, persistent eczema is found without any of these common features and the skill of the herbalist is in tracking down the causes or exacerbating factors. Careful diary keeping is invaluable.

The herbal approach relies heavily on both joint observations with the parents and detailed examination of the child's health. Typically, herbalists look at the skin drainage and consider circulatory herbs (*Myrica, Zanthoxylum, Piper*); lymph drainage of the skin (*Calendula, Burdock*); liver function (*Taraxacum, Rumex, Berberis*); kidney function (*Aphanes, Apium, Galium, Taraxacum, Parietaria*); digestive and bowel function (*Rumex, Acorus, Jateorrhiza, Matricaria, Gentiana*); the nervous system (*Verbena, Tilia, Hypericum, Valeriana, Avena*); the so-called antidyscratics or metabolic stimulants that have particular value in skin diseases (*Echinacea, Viola tricolor, Trifolium, Solanum dulcamara*); and herbs that encourage the body's own steroid production (*Glycyrrhiza, Dioscorea, Smilax*). The diet would be examined in detail and any suspect allergens or intolerances tested, together with a general move to a more 'cooling' and cleansing diet with fresh fruit, salads and less rich, sweet foods as necessary. With children, nutritional composition of the diet is very important and any changes need to be checked with a herbalist or dietician.

Skin creams based on *Matricaria* or *Calendula* help calm the inflammation, or *Stellaria* where there is severe itching. These can be combined with either *Quercus* or *Hamamelis* where there is a weepy eczema. Oat bran can be added to bath water and strong infusions of either *Calendula* or *Matricaria* are very soothing if used to bathe hot itchy rashes or added to the bath water before a comforting soak. Avoid hot baths, which aggravate the rash.

Worms can be a nightmare. Social embarrassment aside, however, they are rarely harmful. Serious or prolonged infections of some species can lower the child's constitution and produce abdominal pains, diarrhoea, and listlessness. Children are most often infected because of their lower interest in toilet hygiene and the close social interaction at nursery and school.

The most common culprits in temperate countries are thread-worms and roundworms. Contrary to popular belief, or perhaps fantasy, the worms are tiny and difficult to see. Threadworms, as their name suggests, are white and threadlike at around 3-10mm in length. They are noticed by the constant scratching of an itchy anus because the female emerges at night to lay eggs on the skin around the opening. Most cases of worms in temperate countries are due to these worms and they are usually harmless.

Roundworms are larger (to 15cm) and less common. They are also found in cats and dogs as well as other children, which means there are more opportunities to catch them. Pet-loving cultures should take care to worm their cats and dogs regularly. These worms also live in the intestine but burrow through the wall and can travel to other organs of the body where they can cause a wide range of problems including blindness.

Tapeworms provide the origin of the idea that worms are very long. This worm is rare in humans as it is caught only by eating uncooked infected pig meat. The worm is indeed like a flat ribbon or tape and can be 3 metres long. The head is permanently dug into the intestine and the tail grows and breaks off in segments which are seen in the stool. These segments are full of eggs but have to be eaten to spread.

Roundworms and threadworms are treated herbally with teas of *Tanacetum, Matricaria,* and *Artemesia*. These should be taken daily for at least six weeks. Garlic cloves, eaten raw in food, and a two-day diet of grated carrot have also been used with efficiency. Carrot is gently laxative, but the tea treatments should be backed up with a gentle laxative given for three days each week for three weeks. The teas weaken the worms, which must then be efficiently expelled from the intestine.

Round worms are more difficult, especially if they have migrated from the gut. The enzyme papain from pawpaw fruit dissolves the outside skin of the worms while in the gut. Lucky people in the tropics can eat fresh pawpaw daily for three weeks, but the unfortunate temperate dwellers must resort to papain in tablet form.

Beware of any of the following symptoms, which may indicate conditions that should be treated by a doctor or herbalist:

- temperature rises to 40°C (104°F)

- constipation lasts four or more days

- diarrhoea lasts more than four days

- diarrhoea occurs with vomiting

- there is difficulty in breathing, with or without a fever

- baby or child is doubled up with distressed crying, feels sick and may vomit

---

SKIN, HAIR AND NAILS

The skin is a tough, actively growing and self-replacing covering of the outside of the body. It differs in structure and function in different places. The skin of the eyelids is thinner and more flexible than that covering the sole of the foot. The skin over the fingertips and lips is more sensitive to most sensations than is that over the knee or scalp. The functions of the skin are impressive. It protects the inside of the body from outside attack by microbes as well as keeping the inside from spilling onto the outside! It is littered with sensory devices to detect the lightest touch, pinpricks, temperature, and pain. It is a reverse raincoat, keeping water in the body, but it leaks sweat in a controlled way to cool the body. In cold weather, the body hairs stand erect to trap more air between the shaft and keep the heat in. The skin also has a mild excretory function, with small amounts of waste being released in sweat. Hair and nails are specialized structures within the skin. For both sexes in most cultures, it has a cosmetic role, which is the least important, physiologically speaking, but is where most human attention is lavished on the skin. Sun-tanning, cosmetic decoration, tattooing, hair and nail grooming, and lavish attempts at preservation absorb large proportions of personal budgets and time. Skin also has a psychologically important function. It is what we present of ourselves to the world.

The skin is also the largest organ in the body and its function and health are closely related to everything else that goes on under the skin. For the herbalist, the skin is the external sign of the body's health. Many serious illnesses of the internal organs or tissues – cancers, Cushing's and Addison's diseases, diabetes, Crohn's, and even vitamin deficiencies – affect the skin. Here we are concerned with the more common skin, hair and nail conditions, but keeping in mind always the close relationships between the inside and outside of the body.

Eczema is one name for the more general term for inflamed skin – dermatitis. The precise cause is not known but there may be some deficiency in essential fatty acids or interference with their metabolism. The rash can take many shapes, appearances, and behaviours. It is typically red, itchy, and scaly, and may have tiny blisters or spots that can weep. Typical eczema is found on the inside of the elbows and the backs of the knees, but can be found anywhere. The one common element is that eczema is a clear case of the skin being a mirror to the internal state of the body.

There are two broad groups of eczemas. The endogenous types are due to changes within the body. The most well known is atopic eczema. Here people develop a 'trigger happy' immune system at an early age and tend to have allergic responses to a wide range of common allergens – house dust, pollen, animals, foods or food ingredients etc. Sufferers usually experience hay fever and asthma as well as other allergies.

Other endogenous forms include varicose eczema and seborrhoea. Poor local circulation is the cause of varicose eczema, usually in the lower legs. The painful, slow-to-heal leg ulcers that are common in the elderly often start with varicose eczema. Reduced blood flow in the legs produces both a red scaly area and vulnerability to infection from the slightest injury. A slight bruise or graze is enough to result in an infection that soon becomes an ulcer. Because of the reduced blood supply, the small infection cannot heal as the body's defences against microbes and its healing powers are carried in the blood. They are slow to heal unless circulation is improved. Seborrhoea includes the slightly scaly, pale pink rash found typically across the forehead, eyelids, top of the chest, or into the scalp. Another minor but common form of endogenous eczema is discoid eczema. Small disc-shaped patches appear, usually in the same spot, and itch to announce their presence. They come and go without treatment and usually are related to stress.

The exogenous eczemas are more directly related to contact with some irritant substance. Washing-up liquid or powders, oils and cosmetics are common chemicals that affect the skin directly, usually on the hands where the contact is first made. Allergic eczemas follow sensitization of the skin by contact with chemicals like dyes, rubber and metals, or with house plants or some animals. The sufferers sometimes find they suddenly become allergic to something they have had no problem with before.

Exogenous eczemas are best treated by identifying the external factors and avoiding them or protecting the body from direct contact with them. The endogenous types, however, are approached by herbalists through improving the body's functioning. Successful treatment relies on a careful and accurate unravelling of both the factors making the condition worse and how the body functions.

The symptoms of scaling and itching can be eased dramatically with light creams (*Calendula, Matricaria, Stellaria*), adding a gentle astringent where there is weeping (*Hamamelis, Potentilla*). Avoid creams with lanolin as an ingredient because it is a common allergen and could make the rash worse. Internally, herbalists could look to digestive function (*Acorus, Gentiana, Jateorrhiza*); liver and bile flow to improve clearing of the blood (*Rumex, Berberis,*

Taraxacum, Urtica, Scrophularia); blood circulation (*Zanthoxylum, Myrica, Zingiber*) and cleansing (*Galium, Urtica, Arctium*); alteratives (*Echinacea, Phytolacca*); adrenal stimulants (*Glycyrrhiza, Smilax*); or nervines to relax and restore a stressed nervous system (*Verbena, Scutellaria, Avena, Melissa*).

Psoriasis can vary from large, thick red plaques with thick white scales of skin to very mild red patches with lighter scaling. It differs from eczema, which is mainly an inflammation of the skin, in being a state of extremely rapid growth (six times normal) of the upper layers of the skin, or epidermis. This is why the areas of psoriasis rash are usually thicker than eczemas, deeper red, and produce such thick scales. The thick form typically develops on the elbows and fronts of the knees. One sign of psoriasis is the presence of tiny pits in the fingernails, but these are not always present. Psoriasis can affect the scalp, groin, palms, and soles of the feet.

The causes are unknown. Psoriasis may run in families and often follows bacterial infections or periods of great stress. Once established, its progress is variable. Some people find it spreads relentlessly whereas others find their rash diminishes and eventually fades only to reappear months or years later. One form is linked to an arthritic condition where the joints are also involved. All psoriasis is difficult to treat, but the arthritic-linked type is particularly resistant.

Herbalists approach psoriasis with a similar strategy to that for eczema. Skin herbs (*Trifolium, Galium, Arctium, Echinacea*) may be combined with liver herbs and especially with adrenal herbs (*Smilax, Glycyrrhiza, Dioscorea*). There may be extensive coverage of both stress and exhaustion of the nervous system (*Verbena, Hypericum, Scutellaria, Elutherococcus, Avena*). Creams can keep the skin moist, which reduces scaling. *Calendula, Matricaria*, and *Hypericum* are generally useful, but an ancient and very effective ointment, that used also to be found in official lists of medicines, is made from *Sambucus* leaves. It used to be known as *Oleum Viridum* or less romantically, as green ointment. It is most effective in combination with three other herbs (*Artemesia, Plantago, Glechoma*).

Impetigo is an infectious bacterial rash of the face and neck. It weeps a clear discharge that dries to a yellowish crust over the redness. It sometimes follows eczema or seborrhoea or even head lice, all of which weaken the skin's defences against bacteria invasion. It is not serious and leaves no scarring.

Herbalists treat the rash with antimicrobial lotions (*Calendula, Thymus, Melaleuca, Thuja*) and treat any underlying weakness in the body or other conditions that may have allowed the infection to take hold.

Acne terrorizes pubescent boys and girls, but can also afflict adults. Many women find a short burst of spots in the week before their periods. The spots are found around the face, especially the cheeks, across the back and sometimes in the 'V' of the neck. Acne can be severe or mild but nearly all sufferers of true acne have, to some degree, blackheads or whiteheads, pustules or 'zits', deep and hard cysts under the skin, and small scars.

The causes are probably varied but all theories include two steps. First an increased build-up of grease or sebum in hair follicles. This is made worse by any change that blocks the escape of this sebum to the outside. Second is the presence of bacteria that live on the sebum and, in the process, release breakdown chemicals that trigger inflammation around the hair follicle. The result is a pustule.

Herbal treatment begins with removing the embarrassment of the spots, cleaning up the skin in the process. One of the best lotions is the anti-inflammatory and antiseptic *Calendula* tincture. This is in 90 per cent alcohol to dissolve the natural resin, which, on drying on the skin, leaves a protective film over the pores and hair follicles. Internal treatment is related to the age and circumstances of the patient. Even in pubescent patients, any aspect of the diet that encourages a greasy skin makes matters worse. As well as reducing all added fats and simple sugars, compensating the reduced energy intake with light and 'cleansing' fresh fruits and vegetables makes for a healthier diet.

Any excess of androgen hormones at puberty will exacerbate

the problem. Herbs can help regulate these hormones (*Angelica sinensis, Vitex, Chamaelirium, Dioscorea*). Maintaining a healthy blood supply and an efficient skin and blood cleaning system is important. A herbal infusion based on a mixture of these herbs is effective in keeping acne under control (*Calendula, Urtica, Arctium, Taraxacum, Rosmarinus, Viola, Trifolium*). This infusion is pleasant to drink and can be taken indefinitely as a general skin and metabolic 'tonic'.

Boils and carbuncles are infections of hair follicles by a bacterium that can live elsewhere on the body, especially in the nose. Carbuncles are deep infections of a cluster of follicles, and are in effect a nest of deep boils.

Herbal approach recognizes that sufferers are usually either run down or have been following a poor diet that has reduced their metabolic potential. The best treatment is internal, aimed at improving diet, strengthening metabolic activity, and removing any hitchhiking source of future infection. The basic treatment is similar to that of eczema. Anti-infectives and immune stimulants could be added (*Echinacea, Baptisia, Elutherococcus*).

Warts are not caused by evil spirits or by handling frogs. They are viral infections, and can take several forms. Verrucas are viral warts that happen to be on the soles of the feet. Genital warts are spread by sexual contact and are caused by the same group of wart viruses that cause cervical and penis cancers.

Herbal treatments are best limited to the application of herbs to the surface of the warts. *Chelidonium* sap is the most effective. It must be fresh and be applied daily for three or more weeks. The sap is bright yellow-orange and dries a dark brown, causing the cosmetically conscious to avoid it. Less visible is tincture of *Thuja*, which is applied undiluted every day. Thin slices of garlic applied to the warts and held in place by a bandage are also recommended, but not for the breath-wary as the garlic oils are absorbed through the skin and appear on the breath.

Cold sores and herpes are the work of two variants of the virus *Herpes simplex*. It is very infectious and most people are infected in childhood. The virus lives in the nerve roots and waits patiently until the immune system is off guard (after stress, physical or mental exhaustion, or any chronic illness), then appears. The name cold sores is because one sign of a run-down immune system is repeated minor infections like the common cold, which is when the crusting blisters appear around the mouth and lips.

Apart from boosting the whole body's functioning and removing all stresses, the best herbal treatment for the cold sores is a lotion or cream based on *Melissa, Melaleuca, Phytolacca*, and *Echinacea*, all of which are antiviral.

Shingles must be one of the most unpleasant skin afflictions. It is due to the virus *Herpes zoster*, which is the same virus that causes chickenpox. Once infected, the virus lurks in the nerve roots until the immune system is off guard, then it travels up the nerves under the skin and leads to painful inflammation around the nerve endings in the skin. The rash begins as small blisters along the line of the distribution of one of the spinal nerves that serve the skin. After a few days the blisters break and the red and very painful rash develops. It is accompanied by depression.

Even when the rash subsides, there can be severe neuralgia, known as postherpetic neuralgia. For some, this discomfort can be greater than the original rash and can last for years.

The outbreak of shingles' rash is usually a sign of a physically or emotionally depleted person. Treatment should start here. Herbs for the rash follow three lines of attack. Stimulating the immune system and use of internal antivirals (*Echinacea, Elutherococcus*), combined with topical creams designed to kill viruses, relieve the inflammation and ease the neuralgia (*Echinacea, Calendula, Matricaria, Gelsemium, Acontium, Lavandula, Atropa*). The postherpetic neuralgia is helped with local anaesthesia creams based on *Acontium* and *Gelsemium*, and internal treatment aimed at the nervous system (*Hypericum, Verbena, Elutherococcus, Rosmarinus*).

Athlete's foot and ringworm are fungal infections of the skin. They are caused by different fungi but have the same causal background. The fungi are highly contagious and normally cannot take a hold unless the immune defences in the skin are damaged or suppressed.

Athlete's foot loves the warm damp conditions around and between the toes. Trainers and high-sided boots keep feet warm and sweaty and invite any infection to stay. Ringworm can be found on any part of the body but it prefers the arms or trunk. The rash is easily identified because it grows outwards, producing a red margin with paler centre as the growing fungus passes by. The effect is like the fairy rings of mushrooms on lawns.

Herbal treatment is with antifungals (*Calendula, Thuja, Melaleuca*), either as creams or lotions. The infection can be healed quickly but attention must also be given to improving general health to resist further infection.

Thrush is one form of the most over-diagnosed health problem of the 1980s, *Candida*. The responsible organism is another fungus. It is found normally in healthy intestines among dozens of other types of bacteria and fungi, which live in a well-organized and beneficial relationship together, and with us. When the immune system is disturbed, the balance among these gut microbes can be disturbed and the *Candida* fungus multiplies without discipline. Women on antibiotic drugs often develop vaginal thrush infections because the healthy bacteria in the gut and the protective bacteria within their vagina have been decimated by the drug. Elderly people, especially denture wearers, also develop *Candida* infections in the corners of the mouth. If the infection is serious, it may also invade the mouth, where it is seen as white threads that can be easily scraped away. The fungus can invade other parts of the body but usually restricts itself to warm, damp places like the groin, underarms, under the breasts, mouth and vagina.

Herbalists treat thrush with infusions, lotions or creams of anti-fungals (*Calendula, Thuja, Melaleuca*) and anti-inflammatories (*Calendula, Matricaria*). Mouth and vaginal infections are most easily treated with infusions of the above herbs, applied as a mouthwash or douche. For persistent internal infection of the vagina, herbalists can make pessaries that contain the same anti-fungals combined with gentle astringents (*Lamium, Hamamelis*).

Dandruff refers to the fine scales of skin floating away from the scalp. This may be normal skin replacement in some cases. The entire body is covered with a constantly growing layer of skin. All day small flakes are floating away as fresh, new layers push up from underneath. The fine layer of 'dust' that accumulates on bed frames under the mattress consists almost entirely of these skin scales. Fungi that live on the oil produced in the hair follicles also cause dandruff.

Some dandruff closely resembles the seborrhoeic eczema that affects the face and chest. The same causes may apply. Food, shampoos and washing-powders, even the washing water itself could be responsible.

Standard anti-dandruff shampoos help in most cases but there is nothing as efficient as finding the cause. Herbal antifungal and anti-inflammatory hair washes are helpful (*Calendula, Melaleuca, Rosmarinus*).

Insect stings and bites are short-lived crises, but no less memorable for that. Bee and wasp stings are the most serious, both because they are common and because they hurt more than the bites of midges, flies or ants.

Bee stings should be scraped off or picked off with tweezers and not rubbed. Rubbing empties the sack of venom into the skin and makes matters worse. The stinging chemicals are acidic and can be neutralized by alkaline rubs. Bicarbonate of soda is excellent but not often carried when the sting is experienced. Otherwise apply lavender oil. Wasp stings are alkaline and should be treated with acidic rubs like vinegar if it is handy. Otherwise reach for the nearest dock, plantain or sorrel leaf, which are acidic. In desperation apply lavender oil which has a comforting anaesthetic effect.

Burns and scalds are common enough in daily life. Serious burns should be taken to a casualty department rather than being treated at home. Slight or minor burns can be treated effectively with simple herbal remedies.

Cool the affected area under running water if possible. Do not break any blisters that form. Cover any broken skin with a non-fluffy and non-sticky covering to stop bacterial infection. Herbal treatments include bathing the area with infusions of *Calendula, Matricaria, Potentilla* or *Hamamelis*. Once dried, light creams of *Calendula, Matricaria* or *Hypericum* will help healing.

Nettle rash (urticaria) and angioedema produce raised weals or swelling anywhere on the body. The weals are recognized by the paler inside with a red margin, looking like red coral islands. Angioedema tends to affect the lips, eyes and throat. Both can appear within minutes of exposure to the allergen. Shellfish, strawberries, nuts, animal dander, drugs like aspirin, and some plants are common causes.

Both conditions are harmless unless the throat is affected with angioedema, which can cause suffocation. The urticaria rash may itch, but usually subsides within twenty-four hours.

The best treatment is to identify and avoid any trigger agent. Herbalists may use antihistamine herbs (*Matricaria, Ephedra*) combined with bitters and digestive herbs to stimulate liver and digestive functions (*Artemesia, Berberis, Aristolachia, Urtica*).

Body lice, fleas, and scabies are more common than social acceptance would allow most people to admit. None is the preserve of the lower social groups. Several types of lice share our space. Head lice inhabit scalp hair. They itch and are best identified by the white egg cases left cemented to the hair shafts. The pubic louse also lives in hair but doesn't like the thicker head hair and aims for the pubic region. Body lice congregate in clothing and can be seen in seams and hems. They can attack any part of the body, which they trespass on to suck blood. Lice are caught by close physical contact with another host.

Fleas were the carrier of the notorious black death or bubonic plague. Today they are mere irritants, biting the feet and legs of inhabitants of and visitors to houses they invade. The human flea is less commonly the culprit than cat and dog fleas. Pets carry the fleas, which drop their eggs onto floors and furniture. The eggs hatch into fleas that jump from the floor onto the legs of any passing source of vibration, in the full expectation that it is a cat or dog on which to feed. They are not discriminating.

Scabies is due to a small mite that burrows under the skin, on which it feeds. Its faeces are also deposited under the skin and cause an allergic reaction, which results in the first symptom, intense itching. This is due to an allergic rash that can cover the whole body even though the mites may be restricted to three or four individuals on one hand. The mites are no more than 1-2mm long and their burrows less than 1cm long, so careful examination is essential. They may be seen in the finger or toe webs, or on the hands or feet. Once itching starts, the carrier often scratches so much that a rash from scratching obliterates the mite's burrow. Scabies is caught from lengthy close contact with another sufferer, as from sleeping in the same bed.

Treatment varies with the parasite but conventional practice relies on extremely strong pesticides that many people wisely choose to avoid. The standard lice shampoos contain malathion or carbaryl. Herbalists recommend essential oils from *Sassafras*, *Thymus* or *Quassia* wood. Good hygiene is not a factor, but once an infestation is noticed, all clothing and bedding should be thoroughly boiled and washed, and it is important that all potential contacts are treated at the same time.

Fleas respond well to deterrence. Onion oil, *Lavandula* oil, and crushed herbs (*Artemesia* spp., *Mentha* spp.) are effective. Regular treatment of pets and vacuuming of the floors and furniture to remove eggs before they hatch are recommended.

Self-treatment of scabies is recommended. The conventional approach requires covering the body, up to the neck, with insecticide lotion. Herbalists are more sympathetic, recommending painting a lotion of *Tanacetum*, *Phytolacca*, and *Thuja* tinctures, which kills the mites. The full benefit has to wait until new skin grows, replacing that containing the mites and their waste.

Beware of any of the following symptoms, which may indicate conditions that should be treated by a doctor or herbalist:

- burns that have broken the skin

- moles that are discoloured or growing

- any new or changing lump in a breast

CHAPTER FIVE

Herbal Medicines

THERE IS NOTHING MYSTERIOUS OR MAGICAL ABOUT HERBAL medicines. They are drugs, the definition of which means they have therapeutic benefits and are used to treat either the causes or the symptoms of illness. However, it is not only the fact that they come from plants that makes herbal medicines of special interest. They also have important characteristics that make them both valuable medicines and specifically different from pharmaceutical drugs.

Before probing deeper into herbal medicines, it is useful to be clear what we are talking about. Herbal medicines are not to be confused with the botanical or culinary definitions of 'herbs'. To a botanist a 'herb' is a soft-stemmed, vascular plant. It excludes trees, shrubs, and mushrooms. Culinary 'herbs' include leafy flavourings (oregano, basil, thyme, sage, etc.), but exclude the spices, nuts and seeds that are also used to flavour food. A 'medicinal herb' can be any member of the plant kingdom, used whole or in part. It includes leafy plants, tree bark, roots, seeds and fruits, ferns, cacti, seaweeds, and mushrooms or other fungi. The current technical term for herbal medicines is 'phytopharmaceuticals', but apart from being rather a mouthful for daily conversation at home, it also is not strictly accurate. So, stick with 'herbal medicines' or just 'herbs', in full confidence that *any* member of the plant kingdom may be included.

Around 40 per cent of all Western pharmaceutical medicines are based on either direct extracts of plants or synthetic copies of chemicals found in plants. Such pharmaceutical medicines containing plant ingredients are not the same as the herbal medicines used by a herbalist, but since the world of plants has contributed to both, the best definition of herbal medicines could be *any medicine that uses plant material, crude extracts of plants or isolates of ingredients from plants*. But, for simplicity, in this book a herbal medicine is the whole plant or any extract as used by a herbalist, whereas any purified extract or isolate or synthetic copy is classified among the pharmaceutical drugs.

Pharmaceutical drugs tend to have a single chemical ingredient (e.g. penicillin, a ß-blocker). Some have two or more ingredients (e.g. Anadin Extra contains aspirin, paracetamol, and caffeine). There may be other minor ingredients to stick the tablets together, flavour the drug or increase its activity. These drugs tend to be designed to have a single action on the body. Hence painkillers, diuretics, or sleeping tablets, because they are single ingredient drugs and are very concentrated, tend to have marked and sometimes serious side effects.

> *Pharmaceutical drugs are single ingredient, highly concentrated, single action drugs that are likely to produce several significant side-effects. These drugs are often made from isolated ingredients of plants.*

Herbal medicines differ in important ways. They may contain hundreds or thousands of natural plant chemicals, of which there may be ten to twenty that are identified as the active ingredients. It is rare for herbal medicines to contain only one or a few active ingredients (*Quercus*, or oak bark and galls, contains only tannins). A single medicinal herb usually has several actions. There may be three to five specific actions in a single herb, depending on the active ingredients present. Thus *Matricaria*, chamomile flowers, contains several volatile oils, flavonoids, coumarins, and xyloglucans, which give the following actions: carminative, antispasmodic, anti-inflammatory, sedative, analgesic, and immune system stimulant. The active ingredients are very dilute, which usually means that any side effects are both minor and rarely noticed.

Herbal medicines contain many ingredients, have several different actions, are very dilute, and tend to have few very mild side effects.

In herbal medicines, there is often an interesting and important interaction among the natural chemicals that makes their combined effect in the body different from that of the purified, isolated chemical in pharmaceutical drugs. For example, in nature, vitamin C and a chemical called bioflavonoids are nearly always found together. Although scurvy among sailors was first treated by giving them lemon juice in their diet, it was later found that vitamin C alone was not nearly as effective as giving it along with its natural accompaniment, bioflavonoids. A similar effect is found with the *Digitalis*, or foxglove, from which the valuable drugs, digoxin and digitoxin, are extracted for treating heart failure. The extracted drug causes poisonings because the therapeutic dose is very close to the toxic dose and as the drug is removed only slowly from the blood, the daily dose given is critical. When the drug is given in the natural plant form, the active ingredients interact with other chemicals in the plant resulting in a more controlled availability in the blood. The result is that only a tenth of the amount of digoxin is needed to produce the same therapeutic effect on the body. Thus poisoning is less likely. In Germany, doctors are rejecting the pharmaceutical drug in favour of the original medicinal herb form.

The action of plant ingredients is often stronger and safer when used in the whole plant form rather than as isolated chemicals.

Pharmaceutical drugs are sometimes held to be superior to herbs because they can be provided in precisely measured doses. This is misleading. The precise measure of a drug in a tablet is not the same thing as giving the exact dose needed by a patient. Every individual's response to an amount of a drug is unique. Not only do different people need different amounts of a drug to get the same therapeutic effect, they may also show different side effects to the same amount of a drug. The recommended dose of a drug is only a rough average discovered in experiments. Some patients need more and some need less. This is why everyone has experienced their doctor increasing or decreasing the dose of a medicine to find the effective dose.

With herbs it is not usually possible to state the exact amount of each ingredient in a sample. The composition of herbs does vary. Different seasons, soil types, amounts of sunshine during the growing season, and even the different stage of a plant's life when it is harvested all affect the composition. Research has also shown that the composition of plants also varies during a single day.

Without analysing each batch of herbs, it is impossible to know precisely how much of each active ingredient is present. But this is not so important. Experience has shown the range of variation of composition and the dosage is based on this average. Because the active ingredients are much more dilute than in pharmaceutical drugs, slight variations in concentration are far less critical with herbs. Herbalists use their drugs in the same way as doctors when deciding the best dose of particular herbs for an individual patient. In fact, the variation of response to any drug between individual patients is probably far greater than the variation of concentration of ingredients in different batches. In short, not having precise amounts of ingredients in herbal drugs is of no real importance.

SIDE EFFECTS

All drugs that have therapeutic effects also have side effects. It is wrong to assume that because herbs are 'natural' they are free from side effects. However, it is normally the case that the herbal side effects are so mild they are not noticed by the patient. The commonest effects include slight nausea, headache, and looseness of the bowels. Some people are sensitive to aspirin and may have a skin rash when taking herbs that contain natural aspirin as methyl salicylate. Liquorice is a valuable herb acting on the hormonal system. If taken for long periods it can lead to a temporary increase in blood pressure in susceptible people. All these side effects are well known to herbalists who discuss them with patients and can usually find alternative herbs that cause no problems.

Pharmaceutical drugs tend to have more and more severe side effects. This is partly due to their high concentration. Common drugs have significant effects. Aspirin can cause stomach irritation or bleeding, spasm of the bronchi in the lungs, and skin rashes. It has been advised recently not to give it to any child under twelve without medical advice. Valium, a commonly prescribed benzodiazepine drug, can cause drowsiness, confusion, jerky muscle movements, amnesia, headache, low blood pressure, rashes, visual disturbance as well as dependence. Another common drug group, the diuretics used in high blood pressure, have side effects that should be taken seriously. They can cause impotence, disturbances of potassium in the blood, alkalosis, raised uric acid, high blood cholesterol, and rashes.

Pharmaceutical drugs can produce more serious effects known as adverse or toxic effects. Around five out of every hundred hospital beds in Britain are occupied by patients ill due to their drugs and while in hospital, twenty out of every hundred patients will be made ill by their medications. Among these adverse effects are heart and blood disorders, hepatitis, adrenal failure and internal bleeding. Common groups of drugs that are the most likely to cause death include digoxin or digitoxin, antibiotics, aspirin,

141

steroids, anticoagulants, and phenylbutazone, which is a potent anti-inflammatory used in hospitals. Doctors are getting increasingly worried about these effects. They have good reason. Modern drugs are more complex chemicals and tend to be stronger in their actions. With more and more of these new drugs being prescribed, it is harder to keep up with any interactions between different drugs, much less know what drugs any patient may be taking.

SAFETY OF HERBS

That herbs are as safe as daily foods is a useful cliché. Most foods when eaten in the amounts normally consumed cause no problem. But many foods (peanuts, strawberries, shellfish, cow's milk, wheat, etc.) produce allergic reactions in some people. The allergic reaction may be no more than a rash but it can cause such swelling of the throat that the airway is blocked and suffocation may result. Other foods contain toxic chemicals, which in higher than normal doses cause illness. Pesticide residues on daily food are of increasing concern. The key issue is the dose.

Most herbs have been used for thousands of years and any serious toxicity would have shown itself already. This could be why so few toxic plants are used medicinally. When herbalists choose herbs for a patient, they are selecting herbs that stimulate natural body functioning to a healthier level, thus reducing or removing the cause of the symptoms of illness. Herbs that were toxic or had severe side effects would produce the opposite of the desired effect and would not be selected. Today's herbal legacy is of countless experiments with herbs in healing and the selection of herbs that are both safe and effective.

The above applies to 95 per cent of all medicinal herbs. There are of course herbs that do have toxic effects. *Atropa, Hyoscyamus, Acontium* and *Digitalis* are valuable herbs that should be used only by qualified herbalists who know when they are useful and what doses are safe and effective.

All herbs are drugs and should be treated with the same respect as any other medicine. Use them only when necessary and only when you know how to use them. If in doubt always consult a herbalist or your doctor.

ACTIVE INGREDIENTS

There is no need to have a university degree in chemistry to appreciate the range of active ingredients in herbs. Of the thousands of chemicals in any plant, there are several groups that have special medicinal value. It is usual that more than one of these groups are found in any one plant. It is the amount of each active ingredient present, as well as the combinations, that determines the medicinal uses of plants. The following is not a complete list of types of ingredient but indicates those that are the most useful in important herbal medicines throughout the centuries. It is worth remembering that there are herbs that have distinct and important medicinal value, without having released their secrets to researchers. As research continues and our understanding of how herbs work expands, then we will be the better able to use herbs in healing.

PLANT ACIDS

The tang of lemons, green apples and sorrel is due to acids. There are thousands of acids in plants where they are probably the most common chemical compound.

The simplest acids include formic (nettle stings), acetic (vinegar) and oxalic (spinach and rhubarb). Succinic and fumaric acids irritate the bowel, making them good laxatives. Fruits are rich in citric, tartaric and malic acids which partly explains why fruits make good natural laxatives.

A special group of acids is the essential fatty acids (EFAs) found as part of the chemical structure of fats and oils in plants. They are more concentrated in the polyunsaturated plant oils. The EFAs have a wide range of functions and it is more their lack that is noticed in skin function, the health of blood and membranes, and in the inflammatory process.

CARBOHYDRATES

There is confusion about the value of these substances. Both starch and household (or cane sugar) are carbohydrates. While the former is a desirable component of the diet, the same cannot be said of sugar. Herbalists are interested in a wider selection of this important chemical group that is a hallmark of higher plants. Green plants produce simple carbohydrates from sunlight, water and carbon dioxide and convert it into all manner of useful substances from wood to the sugar used for energy in the plant.

The pectin used in jam making is a useful laxative as it holds water in a soft gel. The seed coat of a *Plantago* seed contains another gelling carbohydrate that is an excellent bulk laxative. Lactose or milk sugar also works as a laxative but it works differently, by keeping water in the bowel so the stool stays soft.

Mucilage is a slippery, slimy-feeling carbohydrate found in many leaves and roots, notably *Althaea*. It coats mucous membranes in the body, protecting them from irritating substances. It also calms the intestines by protecting the nerve endings in the gut wall from irritants or allergens. The mucilages are soothing to the lungs and urinary systems in dry irritated conditions like asthma or cystitis. These organs are connected with the stomach during their embryonic development. The effect of mucilage on the stomach wall also stimulates a soothing reaction, by reflex or indirect action, on the lining of the lungs or urinary tubules.

PHENOLS

The aromatic ring structure of the chemical benzene provides the building block of this potent group.

Salicylic acid, or aspirin, is a slightly changed version of methyl salicylate. This is the ingredient in willow bark (*Salix*) and meadowsweet (*Filipendula*), both of which have been used for centuries as anti-inflammatories in conditions like rheumatism. It is also in *Gaultheria* or oil of wintergreen.

Phenol itself is a powerful antiseptic and other members of the group are found in antiseptic, antifungal, and antimicrobial herbs, especially among their essential oils (see below). Phenols heat the skin and find a role in rubs and liniments.

Tannins are a diverse group of phenols with one common feature. They all precipitate proteins, which is why they are used to 'tan' leather. The leaves and bark of forest trees, the outside of some fruits and nuts, as well as insect galls, are rich sources. In healing, the tannins form a tough protective layer over damaged or inflamed tissues. They are useful in burns and wounds, and in protecting the gut wall from irritating chemicals. Because they precipitate proteins, they are excellent antimicrobials, because they have the same effect on their proteinaceous cells' walls as they do on animal skins during tanning. Tannins also precipitate alkaloids and have been used to counteract alkaloid poisoning by precipitating the chemical in the stomach and stopping its absorption.

A small group are the coumarins. These are responsible for the smell of new mown hay. They are valuable anticlotting agents.

Anthraquinnones are derived from simple phenols and offer the most dramatic stimulant laxatives (*Rhamnus, Frangula, Cassia*). Milder laxatives based on the same chemicals are found in the dock family (*Rumex*).

Flavonoids and flavones are the sources of many of the yellow colours of flowers. They are bitter (see below), diuretic, antiseptic, and anti-inflammatory. There are many useful chemicals within the group and many plants that may be useful because of other ingredients also often contain flavonoids. The related bioflavonoids are also known as Vitamin P, and include rutin and hesperidin, which are particularly useful in strengthening blood-vessel walls. The milk thistle (*Carduus marianus*) and other thistles contain silimarin, which has the interesting and valuable action of protecting and speeding the repair of liver cells.

VOLATILE OILS

Almost every perfumed smell from plants is due to essential oils. This is a complex group. Each oil is known by its plant source, but these oils are really mixtures of many volatile ingredients. Their chemical structure is based on a small building block called a terpene. Among the simplest volatile oils are the monoterpenes, including pinene, camphor, menthol, limonene, thujone. They are antiseptic, anti-fungal, antiworm, skin-heating, expectorant, carminative and diuretic. Citronellal is strongly repellent of insects.

The sesquiterpenes are more complex. The azulene in chamomile and *Achillea* is a valuable example. It is anti-inflammatory and antispasmodic as are both disabolol and farnesene, which are also present in chamomile.

SAPONINS

Apart from the curious property of forming a lather-like soap, these ingredients are among the most interesting in herbal medicines. There are two groups. One, the steroidal saponins, are similar in structure to hormones and mimic their actions in the body. The other group, the triterpenoid saponins, also mimic hormones but have powerful anti-inflammatory, sedative, diuretic and expectorant actions. They are found in *Elutherococcus, Panax, Aesculus,* and *Glycyrrhiza.*

CARDIOACTIVE GLYCOSIDES

These have a specific action on the heart muscle, increasing both the speed of pumping and the strength of action. The foxglove

(*Digitalis*) is the most well-known example, but herbalists also treasure the benefits of lily-of-the-valley (*Convallaria*) in treating heart failure.

CYANOGENIC GLYCOSIDES

Herbal cough mixtures have a healthy reputation thanks to this ingredient. They are sedative and relaxing to muscles, and are useful as cough suppressants, blocking the cough reflex in dry, irritated coughs. They are found in *Prunus* and *Sambucus*.

GLUCOSINOLATES

The entire cabbage family is recognized by the pungent and hot sulphurous oils they contain. Horseradish (*Armoracia*) and the beautiful meadow weed, shepherd's purse (*Capsella bursa-pastoris*), contain sinigrin or sinalbin, and sometimes both. They are antimicrobial internally but can burn the skin, so only small doses are advised. On the external skin they cause a healing inflammation known as a counter-irritation, which brings healing blood into the area. They are useful in rubs and liniments on sprains and twisted joints, once the initial swelling has gone.

BITTERS

Here is one of the most useful and uniquely herbal ingredients. Many diverse chemicals have a bitter taste. Alkaloids are bitter, as are flavonoids and the monoterpenes and sesquiterpenes. Gentiopicrin from *Gentiana* and *Centaurea* is one of the purest bitters and provides the classic bitter taste. Bitters are stimulants of digestive and liver function. *Taraxacum*, *Hydrastis*, *Berberis*, and *Cinchona* are valued for their bitter ingredients.

ALKALOIDS

The majority of plant ingredients that interest the pharmaceutical industry and have been extracted for drug manufacture come from this group – morphine, strychnine, pilocarpine, atropine and ephedrine. The most fascinating aspect of their value for human health is that no-one has been able to explain satisfactorily their value to the plants in which they are found. They are very bitter and many are toxic, observations that have given rise to the suggestion that they protect plants from predators.

Alkaloids are based on amino acids, the same building blocks as proteins. They are potent chemicals and many are poisons. The group is large and diverse. The most well known members could be the caffeine in tea and coffee, and opium from which the painkilling alkaloid, morphine, is derived.

ACTIONS OF HERBS

Herbs are chosen and combined in prescriptions according to their actions. The actions depend on the active ingredients. Most herbs have several actions and the skill in choosing the right herbs for a particular patient's needs lies in selecting the right degrees of action and the best combination of actions in the individual herbs that make up each prescription. One consequence is that different herbalists may select different herbs for the same patient. Different patients are unlikely to end up with the same herbs, even when they suffer from the same complaint.

Close study of the actions of each herb will improve your skill in self-treatment. You will learn to select a herb for its actions (as a good digestive, or relaxing expectorant, or gentle relaxant etc.), instead of selecting it as a herb for a disease or condition (one for indigestion, for sleeping or for constipation, etc.), which is too imprecise to be successful. Depending on the cause of eczema, for example, you may need herbs that stimulate liver action, encourage a looser bowel and stimulate circulation. This would be more likely to achieve a result than looking for a 'skin herb' that might make a relieving cream but not do much for the eczema.

BITTERS

Herbalists see efficient liver function as an essential for good health. Many illnesses have poor liver function somewhere in their causes and it is no surprise that herbs that stimulate the liver are part of most herbal prescriptions. Active livers produce more bile which also encourages better digestion and the elimination of waste through the bowel. More bile flow also helps flush out the gall bladder reducing the chances of stones forming.

Actions of bitter herbs:

- promote saliva flow

- promote acid release in the stomach

- promote liver function

- promote bile flow (cholagogue)

- relax sphincter (valve) leaving the stomach

- promote pancreatic secretion

- antibiotic

- reduce allergic reaction of proteins

- stimulate repair of gut wall lining

- stimulate white cell production

- increase activity of the sympathetic nervous system

Bitters are 'bitter' and this must not be disguised or the effect will be lost. Bitters are useful in sluggish digestion, constipation, diabetes, skin conditions, chronic inflammations. The importance of the liver to health in general is such that most simple medicines known as 'tonics' contain bitters to stimulate the liver.

STIMULANTS

The popular idea of a stimulant releasing untapped energy or causing improved mental alertness is different from the herbalist's use of the term. Stimulants increase normal functioning of particular organs. Thus there are stimulants of the circulation, of digestion, of liver function, of the adrenal gland's release of hormones, of the nervous system, etc.

Digestive stimulants include the bitters discussed above. *Myrica, Zingiber, Zanthoxylum*, and chilli or *Capsicum* are used for the circulation. *Smilax* stimulates release of the male hormone, testosterone, and *Glycyrrhiza* stimulates the production of the body's own steroids from the adrenal gland. *Rosmarinus* or *Cola* are good central nervous system stimulants.

Herbal stimulation is always done cautiously to encourage the body's systems back to more normal functioning. It should never be done excessively or exhaustion may follow.

SEDATIVES

Herbs that slow down the central nervous system are sedatives. They slow the flow of energy to and from the brain and are useful in controlling pain as well as excessive brain activity, especially when it is unco-ordinated or damaging to health. Sedatives help in insomnia, anxiety or hysteria but are rarely used alone. They are an adjunct to other approaches. For example, a sedative may help the brain rest in insomnia, but not if there is underlying anxiety which should be tackled at the same time.

RELAXANTS

These calm the organs and muscles of the body. Unlike sedatives that focus on the brain, relaxants calm the whole body. They relax tension in the intestines that can cause irritable bowel syndrome, and in the muscles of the neck and scalp, which can cause tension headaches. Over-stimulated organs and tissues benefit from gentle relaxants. Chamomile (*Matricaria*) and *Valeriana* are excellent digestive and intestinal relaxants. *Datura* relaxes lungs, *Hyoscyamus* the urinary tubules, and *Lobelia* or *Lavandula* the skeletal muscles.

ANTISPASMODICS

These are related to the relaxants but are more specific. Muscles sometimes go into prolonged contraction and seem not to be able to relax. Leg cramps are due to such spasms, which can be painful but can also disrupt organ function. Nervous tension can cause spasms in the muscles of the neck and down the spine. Period pains can be due to excessively strong contractions and spasms of the uterine muscles, which cut off the blood supply and result in severe pain. Muscle spasm in the legs, or Raynaud's syndrome affecting the fingers and toes, calls for antispasmodics to relieve the local spasm. *Viburnum, Valeriana*, and *Lavandula* are valuable anti-spasmodic herbs. Many antispasmodic herbs are also used as relaxants.

TONICS

Herbal tonics are not 'pick me ups'. They are designed to produce a healthy state of 'tone' to specific organs of the body. Mucous membrane tonics strengthen the membranes; liver tonics encourage gentle stimulation to congested or sluggish livers; a nervous tonic increases the receptivity of a debilitated nervous system after disease and after emotional or physical exhaustion. Useful tonic herbs include *Hydrastis* for mucous membranes, *Avena* and *Hypericum* for the nervous system, *Chamaelirium* for the uterus, and *Aesculus* for the vascular system.

HYPO/HYPERTENSIVES

Blood pressure can be too low as well as too high. There are many factors that affect the circulatory system and careful diagnosis is necessary to know how to treat it. Control of water loss from the kidneys, the functioning of the heart muscle and the nervous system, and controls on the diameter of blood vessels all have a role. Although the physiology of circulation is now well understood, in around 80 per cent of all cases of raised blood pressure the cause cannot be identified: these cases are given the confusing name of 'essential hypertension'. Herbal treatment is available for all common causes of raised or lowered blood pressure. Excellent diuretics (*Taraxacum* leaf or *Parietaria*), herbs that dilate (*Viscum, Tilia, Crateagus*) or constrict (*Sarothamnus*) the blood vessels, and herbs that affect the heart muscle (*Ephedra, Convallaria, Leonorus, Crateagus, Rauwolfia, Digitalis*) are widely used. **Warning:** do not attempt to treat blood pressure or heart disease without advice from a qualified herbalist or doctor.

DIURETICS

All diuretics increase the flow of urine but they can do this by different means. Diuretics are useful where malfunction of the kidneys changes the composition of the blood, or a weakened heart results in poor control of the amount of water in the body. Herbal diuretics are renowned for their efficiency and safety. Many common foods are also useful diuretics. The best diuretic is *Taraxacum* leaf, but *Betula, Parietaria, Eupatorium purpureum, Collinsonia* are also efficient. Common diuretic foods are celery, parsley, asparagus and the hot drinks, tea and coffee.

CARDIOACTIVES

Throughout history herbal medicines have had a reputation in treating heart and circulatory disease. Today they are important in treating heart failure, angina, irregular heart beat, and high or low blood pressure, blood clots or thrombosis. *Digitalis* or foxglove is perhaps the best known 'herb for the heart', but is not the most used. Others include *Crateagus, Convallaria, Sarothamnus, Urginea, Ephedra, Melilotus,* and *Leonorus*.

STYPTICS AND HAEMOSTATICS

Once an essential household item when men shaved with cut-throat razors, styptics are now used mainly in hospitals or first aid centres. They are however valuable in any first aid kit or home garden. They stop the flow of blood by encouraging clotting. Strong astringent herbs like powdered oak bark (*Quercus*) stop external bleeding, *Equisetum, Plantago, Achillea,* and *Capsella* are used for internal bleeding.

LAXATIVES

Bowel activity matters to herbalists. The elimination of waste is as important as the intake of water and nutrients. Wherever possible the diet should be carefully chosen to ensure a healthy bowel activity. This means high-fibre foods and not sprinklings of bran onto foods. Alas, this is not always possible or enough and the bowel often needs a helping hand.

When constipation strikes, careful attention must be given to the reasons before reaching for laxatives. There are three main types of laxative action. Choose the wrong one for a bout of constipation and matters could get rapidly worse. Simply eating too little food, however high in fibre, will lead to constipation. The most common reason for constipation is too little fibre in a diet of highly refined foods: it's like depriving a skilled craftworker of the tools for the job! However, there may also be spasm, or too little tone, in the muscles of the bowel wall, both of which also lead to constipation.

Laxatives are of four main types. The first simply increases the amount of fibre in the diet, usually by increasing the intake of high fibre foods: beans and pulses generally, root vegetables, whole cereals, dried apricots and prunes, fresh fruits, especially apples and plums. Second are the osmotic laxatives that keep water within the bowel, stopping the stool being dried and hence hardened on its way to the outside world. Next are the bulking laxatives that form soft gels within the bowel. These are large and indigestible and their bulk stimulates movement in the bowel wall to speed the stool on its way. Because it is soft, it is also easy to pass. The fourth are the better known stimulant laxatives that irritate the bowel wall and encourage rapid movement and hence expulsion of the stool.

Herbal laxatives are often incorporated into pharmaceutical laxative drugs. Senna (*Cassia*) and *Cascara* are the best known stimulant laxatives. Bulk laxatives include *Psyllium* husks and *Linum* or linseed. A specifically herbal laxative action is obtained from the action of bitters (*Rumex, Taraxacum, Berberis, Gentiana*), which stimulate bile flow from the liver. Bile itself stimulates the natural peristaltic action of the muscles in the bowel wall and must be fairly described as the most natural of laxatives.

EMETICS

These drugs stimulate vomiting, which can be lifesaving, in certain cases of poisoning. The suitably named American herb, puke-weed (*Lobelia*), or ipec (*Ipecacuanha*) are reliable examples. These herbs are expectorant in very small doses.

ANTIEMETICS

Vomiting is not always welcome. In travel sickness, morning sickness during early pregnancy, or sometimes with headaches, nausea may lead to vomiting. Herbal drugs like *Zingiber*, *Ballota*, and *Mentha* suppress the urge to vomit.

CARMINATIVE

After indigestion, discomfort from wind and associated colic must be the most common digestive complaint. These drugs relieve both. They are usually herbs rich in aromatic oils: *Zingiber*, *Matricaria*, *Cinnamomum*, *Mentha*, *Elettaria*, *Carum*, *Foeniculum*, *Teucrium scorodonia*.

ANTIMICROBIALS, ANTISEPTICS, ETC.

Microscopic organisms cause many human illnesses from the common cold to malaria. Drugs that combat these invaders have specific names although they are often used loosely. Antibiotics, for example, are useful only against bacteria, which is why it is odd when they are prescribed regularly for the common cold or flu, both of which are due to viruses.

So there are antivirals that destroy viruses, antimicrobials that destroy a wide range of organisms, antiseptics that prevent infections, antiprotozoals that kill protozoans (e.g. Giardia, malaria parasites) and antifungals against fungi. The herbal pharmacy offers many choices against most types of micro-organism. *Salvia*, *Thymus*, *Baptisia* and *Commiphora* are antiseptic and antimicrobial. *Melaleuca* and *Calendula* are antifungal, while *Echinacea*, *Melissa*, and *Thymus* are useful against viruses. Herbs offer a unique benefit here. *Echinacea* and Shiitake mushrooms have been shown to stimulate the white cell component of the immune system, thereby improving the body's own defences against micro-organisms.

ANTHELMINTICS

The curse of intestinal worms is not limited to farm animals and four-legged pets. They also inhabit humans. Round worms and threadworms are the most common worm infections in industrial societies, especially among young children. *Thymus*, *Artemesia*, and *Tanacetum vulgare* are the most efficient herbs. Simple foods like pumpkin seeds, garlic and carrots have also been used.

ANTITUSSIVES AND EXPECTORANTS

A cough is a natural reaction to an irritant in the throat or airways. The problem may be mucus from an infection or dust. Sometimes an inflammation of the lining of the airway causes the cough in the vain hope of removing the problem.

A cough to clear the system of some irritant particles or mucus is beneficial and should not be suppressed unless it causes distress. Other coughs may be more frustrating and themselves become irritating without real benefit. An antitussive can stop these unproductive coughs.

Expectorants help soften thick mucus in the lungs or airways and then expel it. They work in different ways. Some stimulate the production of a thin watery mucus that can be more easily coughed out. Others stimulate the tiny hairs or cilia that line the bronchi and provide an escalator to carry dust and mucus out of the lungs where it can be coughed up or swallowed. It is obvious that an expectorant usually relies on coughing to be effective so expectorants and antitussives should not be combined.

Antitussives include *Prunus* and *Tussilago*. Herbal expectorants are varied in action and include relaxing types (*Tussilago*, *Plantago*,

Thymus, Glycyrrhiza, and *Hyssopus*), stimulating expectorants (*Inula, Primula, Urginea, Ipecacuanha*).

ANTICATARRHAL

Often used in close association with the expectorants are interesting herbs that suppress excess catarrh production. All mucous membranes in the body produce catarrh when irritated or inflamed. The most obvious sources of catarrh are the nasal passages and throat during colds. However, catarrh can be produced in the stomach, intestines, and urinary tubules.

Anticatarrhal herbs work by toning and reducing inflammation of membranes. They are useful in conditions as varied as mucous colitis, asthma and glue ear. The best herbs are *Hydrastis, Glechoma, Plantago, Sambucus, Solidago.*

Herbalists see catarrh production as a sign of general metabolic and nervous system disorder. The type of catarrhal condition has to be identified for effective treatment to be designed. Cold conditions produce a thinner, more voluminous catarrh and are associated with slow, stodgy people who usually eat a carbohydrate rich diet and have low energy. The hot types are usually more energetic, even nervy types, and produce thicker catarrh, as manifest in asthma.

DIAPHORETICS

These drugs have a suitably distracting name for societies embarrassed by sweating. They encourage sweating, a natural function that can be very useful in certain diseases. Many infections cause the body to raise its temperature in response. This is an attempt to kill off the invading infective organism. It is therefore a mistake to suppress the mild fevers encountered during colds and flu. Herbalists encourage these fevers and control them with herbs that promote the sweating. Useful diaphoretics are *Sambucus, Tilia, Mentha, Yarrow, Zingiber.*

ANTI-INFLAMMATORY

Inflammation is a healthy process. The redness around insect bites, scalds, or an infected graze or cut shows the body is doing its job through a protective reaction that also aids healing. Clearly out of control inflammation, as seen in Crohn's disease, rheumatoid arthritis and eczema, is not healthy.

Excess or chronic inflammation is tackled first by seeing to the underlying cause where possible, but the symptoms may also need relief. Most of the bitter (see Bitters) herbs encourage the inflammatory process to speed its work of healing. Excellent anti-inflammatory herbs include *Filipendula, Salix, Harpogophytum, Glycyrrhiza, Calendula, Matricaria, Hydrastis,* and *Phytolacca.*

ALTERATIVES

This action has the literal meaning 'to alter'. It has the effect of altering the nutrition and waste elimination of tissues and organs so their metabolic functioning is enhanced to a more normal level. In traditional herbalism, the alteratives are associated with the depuratives, which are plants with the action of cleansing the blood. Both actions are often found in the same plants.

Alteratives are used most in conditions with tissue congestion or reduced immune function. Typical examples are rheumatism, eczema, psoriasis, swollen lymph glands, and tumours of any kind. Herbs are *Arctium, Echinacea, Galium, Rumex, Phytolacca,* and *Viola tricolor.*

UTERINE AND MENSTRUAL

Herbal medicines are well supplied with different actions directed to women's reproductive organs and their functions. In history, herbs known as emmenagogues were used often to encourage menstruation. In fact they are essentially abortefacient and have been used for centuries around the world. A more common problem today is the choice of herbs for pregnant women. Many household herbs and spices can, in large doses, excite the muscles of the uterus and induce miscarriages. Any woman who even thinks she is pregnant should seek the advice of a herbalist before taking any herbal medication, especially during the first three months.

Useful uterine actions of herbs include reducing excess menstrual flow; relaxing uterine contractions and hence easing period pain; increasing pelvic blood flow and lymph drainage to reduce congestion; heal and prevent infections from PID (pelvic inflammatory disease) to thrush; and reduce or eliminate PMT or PMS (premenstrual tension or syndrome). Specific female hormonal balance can be aided by herbs.

Plants used include *Alchemilla, Leonorus, Caulophyllum, Anemone, Cimicifuga, Mitchella, Capsella, Chamaelirium, Vitex, Dioscorea, Lamium,* and *Rubus.*

HORMONAL

The body's fine tuning mechanism is a complex set of hormones that control the presence or rate of actions from the general metabolic rate (thyroid hormones), through water retention (antidiuretic hormone), to the release of an ovum from the ovary (Leutenising hormone). Without these hormones, we are dead. When they are not supplied in exactly the required amounts when needed, the body misbehaves. Many common illnesses are due to such hormone problems.

Many hormones are very similar, chemically, to steroidal saponins found in many plants. Herbal actions either stimulate glands to release hormones or provide look-alike chemicals so the body thinks there is more of the hormone available than the glands are releasing. *Vitex, Smilax, Glycyrrhiza, Serenoa, Dioscorea, Elutherococcus, Panax.*

WOUND HEALERS

The healing, or vulnerary, action must be among the first use of plants discovered by our ancestors. Even in the relative safety of modern housing, food gathering in supermarkets and safer transport, minor wounds are common. Imagine how much more common wounds were for hunter gatherers.

Healing has many components or stages. Antisepsis may be necessary, stopping bleeding, keeping out infections, and encouraging the wound to heal.

Strong antiseptics and styptics are combined in the tannin-rich astringents (*Quercus, Potentilla*). *Symphytum* (comfrey) is a famous wound healer as one of its common names, knitbone, testifies. Here there is mucilage, which dries and binds the edges of wounds together like surgical stitches, as well as an ingredient, allantoin, that stimulates the regeneration of skin and even bone after damage. Many plants are useful wound healers because of their antiseptic oils, blood-dispersing property, anti-inflammatory benefits, or a combination of several useful actions: *Hypericum, Arnica, Chamomilla, Calendula, Hamamelis, Baptisia.*

RUBIFACIENTS

Deep heat rubs contain ingredients with this action. It is heating, which it does by slightly irritating the skin where it is applied. The local blood vessels dilate and more blood rushes into the area. The blood is heating, but it is also healing, which is why rubifacients are applied.

They are useful on sprains, arthritic joints, torn muscles, etc. Many herbs rich in certain essential oils are used, hence their distinctively strong aromas: *Cajaput, Camphora, Rosmarinus, Syzygium, Armoracia, Capsicum*.

DEMULCENTS AND EMOLLIENTS

These are symptomatic treatments but are very efficient and are appreciated when applied. Demulcents protect tissues from irritation and soothe them, whereas emollients soften and protect. Both include mucilaginous herbs (*Althaea, Symphytum, Ulmus, Cetaria, Plantago, Linum, Tussilago*), but also some astringent remedies. Emollients also include heavy ointments, which soften and protect the skin. These may include healing herbs as well as the oily base.

ANTIPRURITICS

After pain, the next most annoying symptom must surely be that itch that won't go away. Antipruritics reduce itching. There are many causes of itchy skin, from liver disease to allergies and stings. The underlying cause must always be sought and treated where relevant, but symptomatic relief is worthy of deep gratitude and is usually easily achieved with herbs. *Stellaria* is the best itch reliever.

ANODYNES

Pain is one of the commonest symptoms and relief is usually wanted immediately. The best approach is sometimes indirect. Headache pain can often be helped by relieving the nervous tension or dilated blood vessels in the brain. Intestinal cramps or colic need antispasmodics and carminatives that help dispel trapped wind. Joint pain in rheumatism responds to anti-inflammatories. There are also herbal painkillers that either sedate or anaesthetize the local nerves. *Aconite* is so effective it can calm the pain of trigeminal neuralgia. Other herbal anodynes include *Gelsemium, Eschscholzia,* and *Piscidia.*

FORMS OF HERBAL MEDICINES

It is sometimes said that one distinguishing feature of herbal medicines is that the whole plant is used. In fact this is often not the case. It is true that parts of plants may be used whole. Whether eating dandelion leaves (*Taraxacum*), an apple (*Malus* spp.), or ginger root (*Zingiber*), only part of the plant is eaten, though the whole of the part is eaten.

Most herbal medicines use only a part of the plant (leaf, fruit, bark, etc.) but even then it is usually only an extract of the part that forms the medicine. The most common way of taking herbal medicine is as a tea or infusion. This is an extract of soluble ingredients in hot water. Cups of coffee and ordinary household tea are made by the same water extract, which is called an infusion. In each case the coffee grounds or tea leaves are not consumed but are thrown away.

Similar extracts are the basis of most herbal medicines used by professional herbalists, or the starting point for manufacturing a wide range of herbal preparations. Alcoholic extracts, like water extracts, are solutions of various ingredients in a solvent; solutions of alcohol and water in this case. Different strengths of alcoholic solution are used depending on the particular ingredients to be extracted. There are two main types of alcoholic extract. A fluid extract is one part by weight of dried herb to one part of alcohol. A tincture is more dilute, usually one part of herb to three or five parts of alcohol. Homoeopaths use herbal fluid extracts in making their very dilute remedies. They call their fluid extract a mother tincture.

There are as many forms of herbal medicine as there are of pharmaceutical drugs. Starting with either a finely powdered herb or an alcoholic extract, infusions, decoctions, creams, ointments, pills, tablets, lotions, liniments, powders, poultices, plasters, bougies, compresses, pessaries, suppositories, etc. can be made.

HERBAL FORMULAE AND PRESCRIPTIONS

It is usual for a herbal medicine to contain several different herbs. Herbalists may prescribe a tea, which is a mixture of carefully chosen herbs to combine the necessary actions for a patient's health. For example, a tea for cystitis may contain antiseptic herbs, a diuretic to encourage flushing of the kidneys, an antihaemorrhagic herb to stop any bleeding from weakened urinary tubules or bladder tissue, and mucilaginous herbs to soothe the inflamed tissues in the bladder or urethra.

Liquid medicines, usually as tinctures, are the most common form of medicine prescribed by herbalists. They are easy to take, but more important, they allow anywhere from three to ten, or more, herbs to be combined. Both the choice of herbs and the amounts of each can be controlled accurately. Care must be taken because some herbal extracts must be kept apart because they can interact chemically and the medicinal effect can be reduced or lost.

The home remedies chapter includes simple techniques for making useful forms of herbal medicine at home.

CHAPTER SIX

Materia Medica

INTRODUCTION TO THE MATERIA MEDICA

THERE ARE PERHAPS 2,000 PLANTS KNOWN TO BE USED AS HERBAL medicines somewhere around the world. Many of these are close relatives and have the same action. Many are different species but have common ingredients and thus common actions. Even where there are several plants that have the same actions, there may be marked differences in the strength of action or in the combinations of actions available in each plant. In short, herbalists around the world are spoilt for choice.

A materia medica is a listing of medicinal material with details of their composition, uses, actions and doses. The list that follows is only a selection of available medicinal plants. It includes a selection of the main herbs used in Western herbal medicine, whether by professional herbalists or by lay users. The herbs included are not restricted to natives of Europe or even the Northern Hemisphere. Medicinal herbs are an important international commodity, which reflects not only the internationalism of modern herbal medicine, but also the identification of the most efficient herbs from around the world.

All of the herbs included are so well and widely used that there is a well-established body of both clinical experience and scientific data on them.

Entries are presented under the following headings:

Latin name and common name. The Latin name is the internationally accepted language of identification. Botanists change plant names often but, because these names are used to identify medicines around the world there is a reluctance to change the Latin names with botanical whim. The family name is given in brackets. Common names vary within countries as well as between. Only the most used two or three common names are included. The herbs are listed alphabetically by their Latin names because of the great variation of the common names. The index at the back of the book can be used to search for herbs by Latin and common names.

Interesting historical or anecdotal points are mixed with a description of each plant and their geographical distribution. Each entry in the materia medica is illustrated by specially commissioned drawings that reflect the character of each herb as well as its medicinally useful parts. These are not intended for identification purposes.

Parts used Only rarely is the whole plant used in medicine. All or most of the medically useful ingredients are usually found in one or other part of the plant. Some plants contain toxins in certain parts but not others and these dangerous parts must be carefully excluded. The parts listed are the most effective for medicinal use.

Active ingredients Plants contain many thousands of chemical compounds whose purposes and interactions are not completely understood. This is further complicated by the high reactivity of compounds in living organisms, which means that the most modern analytical techniques may not be able to identify the precise nature of biological reactions within living material. The list of active ingredients includes those substances that are present in significant amounts and are thought to be involved in their healing actions.

Actions These are the known medicinal actions of the plant. These actions are not always explained by what is known of the ingredients. Many medicines display several actions but it is important to note that these are not a direct guide to the use of a medicine. Herbalists choose combinations of actions in treating a patient's disease or condition. The skill of the practitioner lies in knowing which actions to combine for each patient's condition. A single prescription usually includes more than one remedy.

Medicinal use This lists the main professional use of each herb. It is not intended for use in self-medication. A special home-remedy kit is available on page 289 for home use.

Preparations This is crucial to ensuring that the active ingredients are extracted efficiently, are made available to the body in a form that can be effective in healing, and are convenient to use. Instructions for preparing remedies for domestic use are included in the home-remedy kit.

Dosage The dosage of herbs varies widely according to the medicinal use of the herbs. With the exception of a small number of relatively toxic herbs, the dosage can vary around a safe range. The dose given here is a guide to that range for adults. Only the dose for dried herbs is given. This can be converted to the weight of fresh plant material easily, or used to calculate the doses of tinctures, pills, etc., which are normally prepared from dried material.

The home-remedy kit suggests doses for individual herbs in the kit.

Achillea millefolium

(Compositae)

YARROW, NOSEBLEED, STAUNCH WEED, MILFOIL

The Greek God, Achilles, used yarrow to stop his soldiers' wounds bleeding. It is a common weed of pastures, roadsides and verges, especially on light soils. A native of Europe, although it is widespread in temperate regions. A herbaceous plant, it grows to 30cm (12in.), with angular stems and 7–10cm (2.75–3in.) long, finely divided, green-grey leaves that look like fern fronds. The flowers are small, white, variously tinged with pink, and packed in clusters at the top of the plant. Flowers throughout the summer. Common. Easily cultivated.

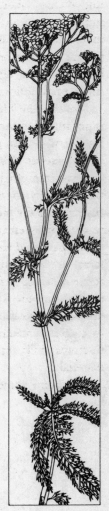

PARTS USED: Whole plant, harvested during flowering.

ACTIVE INGREDIENTS/ACTIONS: Volatile oils such as azulene, which is also in Chamomile; flavonoids, including apigenin and rutin; and tannins. Antipyretic, diaphoretic, anti-inflammatory, astringent, haemostatic and hypotensive.

MEDICINAL USE: A classic fever management herb for flu and the common cold. It is useful in raised blood pressure, especially where the diastolic pressure is raised; for stomach and topical ulcers; it encourages scant or absent periods; and is a good poultice for minor cuts and abrasions. Combines with *Sambucus, Tilia,* and *Mentha piperita*.

PREPARATIONS: Infusions, tincture, poultices.

DOSE: 1–5g dried herb equivalent three times per day.

Acontium napellus

(Ranunculaceae)

ACONITE, MONKSHOOD, BLUE ROCKET, WOLF'S BANE

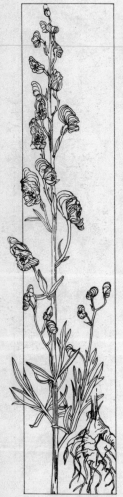

A native of central and southern Europe. There is evidence that it was brought to Britain in pre-Anglo-Saxon times and it can be found wild in the west of Britain. It used to be used as an arrow poison, from which the Latin name is derived. A common and highly poisonous garden perennial. Stems rise to 60cm (24in.) high, with dark-green, deeply divided leaves, and characteristic, deep blue-purple flowers on a spike. Easily cultivated.

PARTS USED: Dried root, collected in the autumn.

ACTIVE INGREDIENTS/ACTIONS: Alkaloids including aconitine and traces of ephedrine and sparteine. Sedative, painkiller.

MEDICINAL USE: It is very poisonous to the heart and central nervous system so is rarely used internally. It is used topically to relieve pain in bruises, sciatica, rheumatism, peripheral neuralgia and lumbago. Never apply it to broken skin. It combines with *Hamamelis*.

PREPARATIONS: Tincture, lotion. Its sale and professional use is restricted by law in the UK.

DOSE: For professional use only.

Agathosma betulina

(Rutaceae)

BUCHU LEAVES, BUCCO, DIOSMA

A small and highly aromatic shrub that is native to Cape Province in South Africa. The Hottentots used it as a body perfume. The pale green leaves are 1.5–2cm (0.5–0.75in.) long and are rounded with a curved point and a leathery feel. Oil glands can be seen on the surface. Flowers are small and white.

PARTS USED: Dried leaves, collected during flowering.

ACTIVE INGREDIENTS/ACTIONS: Volatile oil containing diosphenol, pulegone, and limonene; flavonoids such as rutin, hesperidin, and quercetin; tannin. Diuretic, urinary antiseptic.

MEDICINAL USE: In cystitis, arthritis and prostatitis but should not be used where there is kidney infection. Combines with *Althaea* which soothes a painful urinary tract.

PREPARATIONS: Infusion, tincture.

DOSE: 2–4g dried leaf or equivalent three times daily.

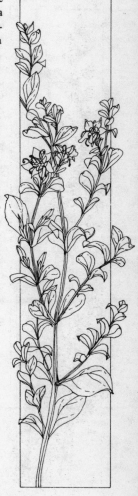

Agrimonia eupatoria

(Rosaceae)

AGRIMONY, COCKLEBUR, STICKWORT, CHURCH STEEPLES

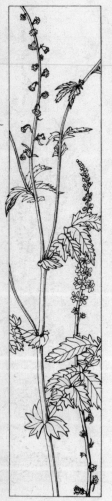

Used for stomach complaints throughout history. One ancient recipe had it mixed with frog's and human's blood to stop internal haemorrhages. The herb tastes so pleasant it is a popular tisane in France. Agrimony grows wild all over Europe, Asia and North America especially on dry waste ground. It has attractive, hairy, pinnate leaves clustered at ground level and a flowering spike rising to 1m (3ft.) in summer. Bright yellow flowers cling to the spike and become cap-like fruits covered in tough hairs which stick to passing animals or clothes. It is easily cultivated.

PARTS USED: Stems and leaves.

ACTIVE INGREDIENTS/ACTIONS: Tannins; coumarins; volatile oil; and flavonoids including apigenin and quercetin. Astringent and diuretic.

MEDICINAL USE: Is a mild astringent that is particularly safe and useful against diarrhoea in children and in mucous colitis. It makes an excellent poultice for ulcers and slowly healing wounds. A gargle for sore throats due to infection or irritation.

PREPARATIONS: Infusion, tincture, poultices.

DOSE: 2-8g dried herb equivalent three times daily.

Agropyron repens

(Graminae)

COUCH GRASS, TWITCH GRASS, TRITICUM, DOG'S GRASS

A noxious garden weed distributed around the world. A native of Europe, it travelled with early explorers and settlers. The name 'couch' may have come from the old Anglo-Saxon word for 'vivacious'. The rhizomes (underground stems) have been used as medicine since the Greek herbalist, Dioscorides. Sick dogs and cats eat the leaves to produce a healing vomit. Culpeper said 'an acre of [couch] to be worth five acres of carrots twice told over'. Smooth white rhizomes spread as a dense network in the soil and produce clumps of grass blades about 10cm (4in.) high. In midsummer a flowering spike appears with two rows of closely packed small flowers, looking like rye.

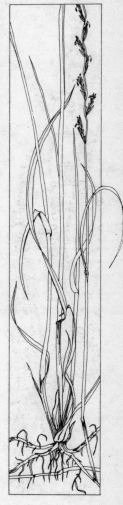

PARTS USED: Rhizome, collected in the spring before the growth spurt.

ACTIVE INGREDIENTS/ACTIONS: A polysaccharide, triticin, and other carbohydrates including inositol, mannitol and mucilage; a volatile oil, agropyrene. Soothing diuretic and demulcent.

MEDICINAL USE: Used mainly in painful urinary tract conditions with inflammation including cystitis, urethritis, and prostatitis. A component of many cystitis tea mixtures.

PREPARATIONS: Infusion, tincture.

DOSE: 1–5g dried herb equivalent three times a day.

Alchemilla vulgaris

(Rosaceae)

LADY'S MANTLE, LION'S FOOT, BEAR'S FOOT

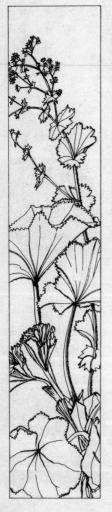

A native of Britain and northern Europe. It is named lady's mantle after the lace collars of women's garments. A perennial with beautiful, lobed, polygonal leaves with fine-toothed margins. Petioles or leaf stalks 15–30cm (6–12in.) high arise from a short stem. Soft, short hairs cover the leaves and stems. From early to midsummer tiny yellow-green flowers appear in clusters on long stalks. Cultivation is easy from root cuttings or seeds.

PARTS USED: Leaves during flowering.

ACTIVE INGREDIENTS/ACTIONS: Tannins. Astringent and styptic.

MEDICINAL USE: Taken internally for diarrhoea and menorrhagia; as a douche for leucorrhoea and vaginal pruritis; as a mouthwash for bleeding gums; and as a gargle for laryngitis or pharyngitis.

PREPARATIONS: Infusion, tincture.

DOSE: 1–5g dried herb equivalent three times a day internally and 30g per litre for douches.

Allium sativum

(Liliaceae)

GARLIC, POOR MAN'S TREACLE

Garlic is one of the few universal culinary and medicinal herbs. Its origins have been lost in history. A native of southern Europe and Siberia. The pharaohs of Egypt and the ancient Greeks and Romans used it regularly as medicine. Culpeper said it was 'a remedy for all diseases and hurts'. The medicinal properties of garlic have been confirmed in many scientific studies. The leaves, which are flat and thin on an unbranched stalk, grow 20-30cm (8-12in.) high. A spherical flower-head of tiny greenish-white or pink flowers appears in July or August. The bulb comprises 8-15 segments or cloves. It is easily cultivated from cloves or seeds.

PARTS USED: Cloves.

ACTIVE INGREDIENTS/ACTIONS: Volatile oil containing sulphur compounds, especially allicin and aliin; geraniol, linalool; flavonoids. Antiseptic, expectorant, diaphoretic, antiviral, anthelmintic, hypotensive, hypocholesterolaemic.

MEDICINAL USE: A traditional remedy for coughs, colds, bronchitis, and respiratory catarrh. Regular use helps prevent colds by strengthening the immune system; it helps lower both raised blood pressures and blood cholesterol.

PREPARATIONS: Fresh cloves; tablets of powdered garlic; dry extracts or capsules of oil; tincture or syrups.

DOSE: 3-5 fresh cloves two or three times a day.

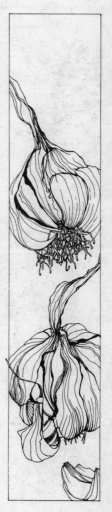

Aloe vera

(Liliaceae)

ALOES, CURACAO, SOCOTRINE

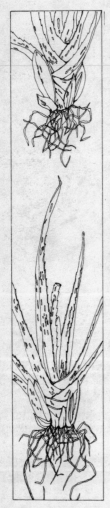

A common ingredient in modern cosmetic skin preparations, but with an ancient pedigree. Aristotle had Alexander the Great studying how the Socotra islanders extracted Aloe juice in 325 BC. A large plant family with more than 200 varieties used commercially, especially those native to east and west Africa. It was introduced to the West Indies in the seventeenth century and is still a major agricultural crop there. The plants have whorls of thick fleshy leaves, usually with a toothed margin, and often without a significant stem. A tall flower spike bearing trumpet-shaped yellow or red flowers appears in the summer. It is easily grown in pots or gardens.

PARTS USED: Juice from the leaves.

ACTIVE INGREDIENTS/ACTIONS: Anthraquinone glycosides (known as aloin), especially barbaloin and isobarbaloin; aloe-emodin; sterols; saponins; resin. Internally, a strong purgative; externally, the fresh juice is an emollient and wound healer.

MEDICINAL USE: The dramatic purgative action is usually made more tolerable by combining it with antispasmodics like Belladonna to stop griping. The fresh juice applied directly to burns, slow-healing wounds, and inflamed skin soothes, protects and aids healing.

PREPARATIONS: Dried powder or tablets, creams, fresh juice.

DOSE: 200-300mg fresh juice to purge.

Althaea officinalis

(Malvaceae)

MARSH MALLOW, GUIMAUVE, MALLARDS, SCHLOSS TEA, MORTIFICATION ROOT

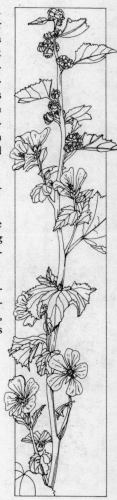

As with many plants it has been both a food and medicine. The Bible as well as both Arab and Chinese literature refer to its value as a food in famines. Manioc in West Africa continues this tradition. It is widely used in European folk medicine. There are many species around the world, especially in the tropics. *A. officinalis* is a perennial shrub growing to 1m (3ft.) high with soft, pale green, lobed leaves about 5 to 8cm (2–3.25in.) long. Unlike other common mallow species, it is covered in soft down. Pale pink flowers, about 4cm (0.5in.) in diameter, with 5 petal clusters in the leaf axils during late summer. The root is thick and tapering. Cultivation is easy from seed.

PARTS USED: Roots collected in the autumn from 2-year-old plants, and leaves collected during flowering.

ACTIVE INGREDIENTS/ACTIONS: Polysaccharide mucilage (20–35 per cent); pectin; flavonoids (in leaves) including quercetin, kaempferol; salicylic acid. Demulcent, emollient, expectorant, and a wound healer.

MEDICINAL USE: It is useful in respiratory catarrh, bronchitis, irritating coughs, gastritis, peptic ulcers, and in urinary tract infections and inflammations including cystitis, urethritis. Locally it makes a good drawing poultice for boils and carbuncles, and a healing one for varicose and other ulcers.

PREPARATIONS: Infusions, decoctions, tinctures.

DOSE: 4–10g dried herb equivalent three times a day of leaf or root.

Anemone pulsatilla

(Ranunculaceae)

PASQUE FLOWER, WINDFLOWER, MEADOW OR PRAIRIE ANEMONE, EASTER FLOWER

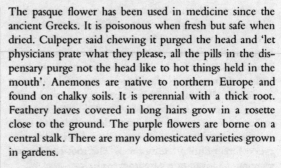

The pasque flower has been used in medicine since the ancient Greeks. It is poisonous when fresh but safe when dried. Culpeper said chewing it purged the head and 'let physicians prate what they please, all the pills in the dispensary purge not the head like to hot things held in the mouth'. Anemones are native to northern Europe and found on chalky soils. It is perennial with a thick root. Feathery leaves covered in long hairs grow in a rosette close to the ground. The purple flowers are borne on a central stalk. There are many domesticated varieties grown in gardens.

PARTS USED: Dried herb.

ACTIVE INGREDIENTS/ACTIONS: Protoanemonin in the fresh herb (which converts to anemonin on drying); saponins; volatile oil; tannins; resin. Sedative, analgesic, spasmolytic, bactericidal.

MEDICINAL USE: Relieves nervous-tension-related and other painful conditions of male and female reproductive systems (dysmenorrhoea, orchitis, prostatitis). Also used in tension headache, hyperactivity, insomnia, nervous exhaustion, and earache.

PREPARATIONS: Infusion or decoction, tincture. **Warning:** Fresh plant should not be used.

DOSE: 0.5–2g dried herb equivalent three times daily.

Angelica archangelica

(Umbelliferae)

ANGELICA

The crystallized stems are found in crystallized peel and confectionery and it is used to flavour liqueurs such as Chartreuse and vermouth. Native to Syria and brought to Europe around 1550, where it may have been important in pagan festivals. In the fifteenth century it was used against the 'plague and all epidemical diseases.' It was seen as a contemporary 'cure all'. Culpeper recommended it for anything from ague to dog's bite and gout. It is biennial, with a thick, fleshy root. The 1m (3ft.) high stems are green and hollow with large dentate leaves. In the second year, large spherical umbels of greenish flowers are produced in September to October. It has a characteristic and strong smell. Cultivation from seed is easy.

PARTS USED: Dried roots and seeds, fresh or dried leaves and stems.

ACTIVE INGREDIENTS/ACTIONS: Volatile oils in the roots and seeds include pinene, borneol, and linalool; valerianic acid; coumarins; iridoids; resin; tannins; bergapten. Spasmolytic, diaphoretic, expectorant, bitter, carminative and diuretic.

MEDICINAL USE: Catarrh and bronchitis; flatulent dyspepsia; digestive stimulant and liver tonic.

PREPARATIONS: Infusion, tincture.

DOSE: 0.5–3g dried herb equivalent three times daily.

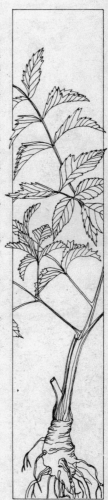

Arctium lappa

(Compositae)

BURDOCK, BEGGAR'S BUTTONS, GYPSY'S RHUBARB, LOVE LEAVES, CLOT BUR

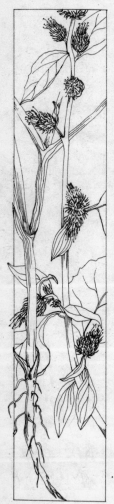

One of the most used European herbs, best known now in dandelion and burdock soft drink. The Japanese use the roots as a vegetable for the dietary fibre. Shakespeare mentions it in three plays. A native of northern Europe but found in Asia and North America. Culpeper said it was so well-known 'even by the little boys, who pull off the burrs to throw at one another, that I shall spare to write any description of it.' For the less familiar, it is perennial and grows to 1m (3ft.), with large arrow-shaped leaves and thistle-like purple flowers surrounded by tiny hooks which stick to passing animals. The deep tap root can grow to 2m (6ft.).

PARTS USED: Leaves, seeds and root.

ACTIVE INGREDIENTS/ACTIONS: Inulin in the root; polyacetylenes in the root; lignans including arctigenin; sesquiterpenes in the leaves; fixed oil; organic acids including phenolic acids. Diuretic, alterative, lymphatic, orexigenic, antibacterial, and aperient.

MEDICINAL USE: Widely used for skin diseases, especially eczema and psoriasis, but also for boils and carbuncles. Useful in gout and rheumatism and as an mild appetite stimulant in anorexia. Helps in cystitis.

PREPARATIONS: Infusion, decoction, tinctures.

DOSE: 2-10g dried herb equivalent three times daily. It is best to start with a small dose and increase that slowly.

Arctostaphylos uva-ursi

(Ericaceae)

BEARBERRY, UVA URSI, HOGBERRY, BEARGRAPE, SANDBERRY

The Latin name comes from the Greek for bear's grape. Used as a diuretic in Europe since the Middle Ages. Its antibiotic action was approved by German physicians in the eighteenth century. The diuretic ingredient, arbutin, passes through the kidney unchanged so its action can be exerted along the urinary tubes. It grows throughout the northern hemisphere at high altitudes and is also found in North America, Europe and Asia. The plant is low and creeping with ovoid or spatula-like leaves 1-2cm (0.4-0.75in.) long and small clusters of white or pink, waxy flowers. It is strongly aromatic.

PARTS USED: Leaves collected in late summer.

ACTIVE INGREDIENTS/ACTIONS: Hydroquinones including arbutin; iridoids; flavonoids including quercetin; tannins; volatile oils; ursolic acid. Diuretic, antiseptic, astringent.

MEDICINAL USE: Used in cystitis, urethritis, dysurias, pyelitis and prostatitis.

PREPARATIONS: Infusion, tincture and tablets.

DOSE: 1-5g dried herb equivalent three times daily.

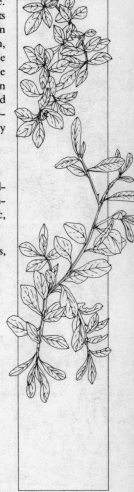

Armoracia rusticana

(Cruciferae) also known as *Cochleria armoracia*

HORSERADISH, RED COLE, MOUTADE DE ALLEMANDS, GREAT RAIFORT

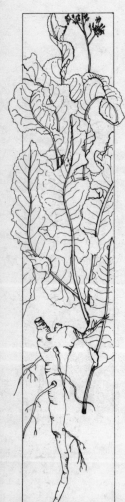

The same flavouring that disguises the blandness of over-cooked beef and which the herbalist Parkinson said, in 1640, was 'too strong for tender and gentle [British] stomachs'. The Germans use as the French use mustard. A robust native of central and eastern Europe but naturalized in many temperate countries and found as a garden escape. The leaves are long and tapering to 1.5m (4.9ft.), growing from a tap root to 70cm (27.5in.) deep. A 90cm (36in.) tall flowering raceme with bunches of white flowers appears in late summer. Easily cultivated but becomes feral easily.

PARTS USED: Freshly harvested roots.

ACTIVE INGREDIENTS/ACTIONS: Glucosinolates, mainly sinigrin, which combine with water when crushed, producing the aromatic and pungent mustard oils; Vitamin C; resin. Stimulant, diuretic, diaphoretic, rubifacient, and antibacterial.

MEDICINAL USE: A powerful circulatory stimulant. The mustard oil is antibiotic and is useful in infections of the lungs and bronchi. It has been used topically in gout and rheumatism.

PREPARATIONS: Freshly grated root used as poultices; syrups; tincture. Care is necessary with the poultice as the plant may cause blistering.

DOSE: 2-5g dried herb equivalent three times daily.

Arnica montana

(Compositae)

ARNICA, LEOPARD'S BANE, WOLF'S BANE, MOUNTAIN TOBACCO

The most famous bruise and wound remedy. Has been used since the sixteenth century. The German poet, scholar and statesman, Goethe, claims it saved his life after a serious fever. Native of central Europe, especially in mountain pastures. It is perennial with a creeping rhizome sending up a rosette of small downy leaves in the first year. A tall stem with few leaves but large, orange, daisy-like flowers rises in the summer of second year. Cultivation best by root division in spring.

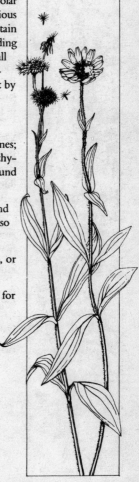

PARTS USED: Flowers and root.

ACTIVE INGREDIENTS/ACTIONS: Sesquiterpene lactones; flavonoids; methylated flavonoids; volatile oil with thymol; arnicin (a bitter); mucilage. A counter irritant, wound healer, vasodilator, phagocytosis stimulant.

MEDICINAL USE: An effective application for bruises and sprains, even for chilblains, where skin in unbroken. Also for alopecia neurotica.

PREPARATIONS: Tincture, homoeopathic preparations, or creams.

DOSE: Use tincture externally only. **Warning:** Not for internal use.

Artemesia absinthium

(Compositae)

WORMWOOD, GREEN GINGER, ABSINTHE

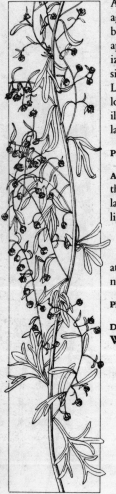

An ancient household strewing herb against insects and against clothes moths. It has been used instead of hops in brewing and is an ingredient of liqueurs (absinthe) and aperitifs (vermouth). Native to Europe and is now naturalized in North America. It grows freely on untended roadsides and on wasteland. A perennial with firm, leafy stems. Leaves are pale from thick downy hairs, are 5cm (2in.) long and deeply cut with blunter ends than the closely similar mugwort (*A. vulgaris*). Small yellow flowers appear in late summer. Easily cultivated and propagated vegetatively.

PARTS USED: Dried herb harvested during flowering.

ACTIVE INGREDIENTS/ACTIONS: Volatile oils containing thujone, azulenes, bisabolene, pinene, etc.; sesquiterpene lactones; flavonoids including quercetin; phenolic acids; lignans. A bitter, stomachic, choleretic, anti-inflammatory, and anthelmintic.

MEDICINAL USE: A stimulating digestive in anorexia, atonic gastritis. Effective against parasitic worms and nematodes.

PREPARATIONS: Infusion, tincture.

DOSE: 0.5–2g dried herb equivalent three times daily. **Warning:** Not to be taken for extended periods.

Atropa belladonna
(Solanaceae)

BELLADONNA, DEADLY NIGHTSHADE, DEVIL'S CHERRIES, DWALE, DEVIL'S HERB

Folklore has it that the devil nurtures the growing plant. Its alkaloids are among history's most employed poisons. Duncan I of Scotland had Macbeth's soldiers present the invading Danish army with a gift of liqueur doctored with *Atropa* extract during a truce. The Danes drank gratefully, slept and were murdered in their comatose sleep. The name 'belladonna' comes from the cosmetic tradition of Italian women, who used the plant to dilate their pupils, which made them even more sexually appealing. *Atropa* is not to be confused with woody nightshade, which is the same family but a very different plant in all respects. *Atropa* is native to southern Europe but found in Asia, north Africa and North America. A perennial to 2m (6ft.), with dull, ovate leaves from 6-20cm (2.4-8in.). Purple, bell-shaped flowers appear in summer, followed by large 2cm (0.75in.) black-berries nesting on a large calyx. All parts of the plants are poisonous, especially the berries. Cultivation from seed.

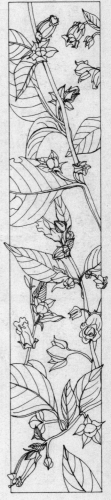

PARTS USED: Herb and dried root.

ACTIVE INGREDIENTS/ACTIONS: Tropane alkaloids including hyoscyamine, atropine; flavonoids. Narcotic, sedative, mydriatic, antispasmodic.

MEDICINAL USE: Useful in severe intestinal, renal, or gall bladder colic; in excessive salivation or sweating; and in bronchial conditions such as asthma. It has been used topically for rheumatic pain. Side effects include palpitations, raised blood pressure and intense thirst. **Warning:** Not to be taken except under supervision of a qualified medical herbalist.

PREPARATIONS: Infusion, tincture or cream.

DOSE: To be used only on a qualified herbalist's prescription.

Avena sativa

(Graminae)

OATS, GROATS

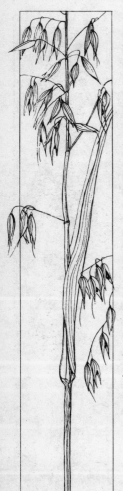

Oats is less important as a food staple than all other cereals because it lacks the nutritional quality. Samuel Johnson appreciated this and said oats was 'A grain, which in England is generally given to horses, but in Scotland supports the people'. Its origin is unknown but it has probably been eaten, if not cultivated, since Neolithic times, and certainly was grown in Europe in the Bronze Age. It has also been used widely in medicine. Its traditional uses as a general nutritive and nervine have been confirmed by recent experiments. An annual grass easily distinguished from wheat or barley by the loose flowering head and the papery covering of the grains. Wild oats varieties are naturalized escapees from ancient fields.

PARTS USED: The flowering tops.

ACTIVE INGREDIENTS/ACTIONS: Alkaloids; flavonoids; protein; minerals including silica and calcium; vitamin E. Nervine, mood enhancer, trophorestorative for nervous system, emollient.

MEDICINAL USE: Useful in nervous exhaustion, depression, melancholia and generally for debility involving the nervous system, especially conditions like shingles, multiple sclerosis, or herpes.

PREPARATIONS: Groats, oatmeal, oatbran, whole plant juice, tincture.

DOSE: Two or more servings of oatmeal per day or 2-5g dried herb equivalent three times daily.

Balotta nigra

(Labiatae)

HOREHOUND, HOARHOUND, BLACK STINKING HOREHOUND

As the common name suggests, this is a bitter-tasting herb. The generic name, which is Greek for 'reject', hints at the tendency of grazing animals to ignore this plant. Culpeper classified hoarhound under the planet Mercury and used it to 'cure the bites of mad dogs'. A native of temperate, eastern Europe from where it spread with population movements across Europe and beyond. It grows in road-side ditches, hedgerows and other moist waste places. As with all members of the family *Labitae*, stems are square and hairy with creeping roots. Heart-shaped leaves 2-5cm (0.75-2in.) have scalloped edges and small purple, lipped flowers in their axils from late summer. Readily cultivated but its enthusiasm may be a problem.

PARTS USED: Flowering tops.

ACTIVE INGREDIENTS/ACTIONS: Flavonoids. Antemetic, sedative, antispasmodic, expectorant.

MEDICINAL USE: For all nervous or hormonal causes of nausea and vomiting, especially in pregnancy, and also in nervous dyspepsia.

PREPARATIONS: Infusion, tincture.

DOSE: 2-5g dried herb equivalent three times daily.

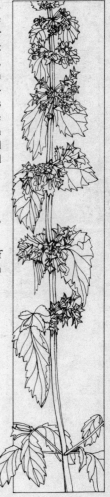

Berberis vulgaris

(Berberidaceae)

BARBERRY, PIPPERIDGE BUSH

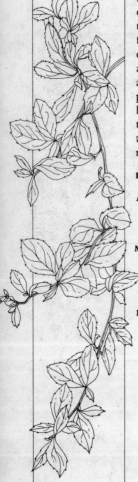

Although indigenous to Europe, it was declared the farmers' enemy in the nineteenth century because it harboured the wheat rust fungus and spread it to each year's new crop from the adjacent hedgerows. It is naturalized in parts of eastern North America. It was encouraged around fields and villages for its fruit from which were made pickles and, according to Mrs Beeton, 'dry sweet-meat, and sugar-plums or comfits'. The deciduous shrub 2-3m (6-9ft.) tall has clusters of four oval leaves protected by three spines at their base. Flowers are small and yellow, appearing in clusters from spring to midsummer and are followed by oblong red berries with a strong acid taste.

PARTS USED: Bark of stems and root.

ACTIVE INGREDIENTS/ACTIONS: Alkaloids including berberine, oxycanthine; chelidonic acid; resin; tannins. Cholagogue, digestive tonic, antibacterial and amoebicidal.

MEDICINAL USE: Used in obstructive jaundice, gall stones, digestive problems with liver involvement following drug or alcohol abuse. For amoebic dysentery and malaria. Avoid in pregnancy.

PREPARATIONS: Decoction or tincture.

DOSE: 0.5-4g dried root equivalent three times daily.

Calendula officinalis

(Compositae)

MARIGOLD, RUDDLES, MARYGOLD, FIORE D'OGNI MESE

A native of southern Europe but familiar around the world as a yellow or orange ornamental plant. The Latin name comes from this habit of flowering on the 'calends' of nearly every month. It has long been used in Indian, Arabic and Greek medicine and remains one of the most useful medicinal herbs, especially for home use. Enormous quantities were grown in Russia, where it was nicknamed 'Russian penicillin'. An annual with angular green stems to 50cm (19.7in.) with resinous and soft-haired, oblong leaves from 5-15cm (2-6in.). Large yellow or orange daisy-like flowers are produced from early summer until the first frosts.

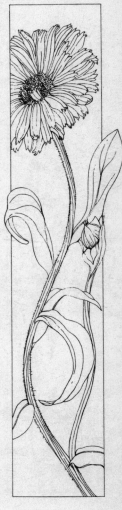

PARTS USED: Flower-heads, leaves.

ACTIVE INGREDIENTS/ACTIONS: Triterpenes; carotenoids; saponins; flavonoids, including quercetin and rutin; volatile oil; resin; chlorogenic acid. Styptic, anti-inflammatory, anti-spasmodic, vulnerary, antiseptic, antifungal, emmenagogue.

MEDICINAL USE: Used internally for conditions where the lymph nodes are swollen, for mouth ulcers, damaged or ulcerated stomach lining, as a gargle for throat infections and oral thrush. Used topically for varicose and crural ulcers, sore nipples, haemorrhoids, anal fissures, cradle cap, eczema. Excellent douche or cream against vaginal thrush.

PREPARATIONS: Infusion, tincture, creams.

DOSE: 1-10g dried herb equivalent three times daily.

Cannabis sativa

(Cannabinaceae)

CANNABIS, GANGA, GUAZA, HEMP, HASHISH, NASHA

Well established in Indian and Chinese medicine for more than 1,500 years, cannabis was brought to Europe by Napoleon after his Egyptian exploits. The drug is a by-product of cultivation of hemp for fibre from which string, sacking and ropes are made. Now better known as a popular, but illegal, narcotic drug. Medical research has shown it valuable as an anti-emetic in chemotherapy for cancer, and as an antidepressant. Cultivated in China, India and southern Russia. Wild plants are common in temperate Europe and North America as escapees from imported birdseed or coarse-fishing bait. An annual growing to 5m (16.5ft.) with beautiful palmate leaves made up of 5–10 long, deeply serrated leaflets. Separate male and female plants bear small and unstriking flowers in late summer.

PARTS USED: Leaf, resin.

ACTIVE INGREDIENTS/ACTIONS: A resin comprising more than 60 components called cannabinoids; volatile oil; flavonoids. Antispasmodic, anti-emetic, narcotic, cerebral sedative, analgesic.

MEDICINAL USE: Used in neuralgia, spasmodic cough and migraine. Used in the United States for relief from nausea in cancer patients on chemotherapy.

PREPARATIONS: Resin or dried leaf for smoking, tincture.

DOSE: Illegal to possess or use without special licences.

Capsella bursa-pastoris

(Cruciferae)

SHEPHERD'S PURSE, RATTLE BAG, MOTHER'S HEART, LADY'S PURSE, STRANGURY

The small heart-shaped fruits resemble both hearts and the purses that used to hang from belts in medieval Europe. Like other successful weeds, it has spread efficiently from its native Europe to all temperate parts of the world. A traditional medicine for stopping bleeding 'inside and out'. Found in light, rich soils. A low-growing annual herb with irregular pale green, hairy leaves 5-15cm (2-6in.) long. A smooth flowering stem rises from the crown, with small, inconspicuous, white flowers emerging from the stem as it grows upwards. Flowering is all year. Readily cultivated.

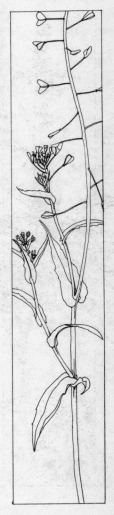

PARTS USED: Flowering herb.

ACTIVE INGREDIENTS/ACTIONS: Flavonoids; polypeptides; fumaric and bursic acids; histamine, tyramine tr., choline and acetylcholine; mustard oil. Anti-haemorrhagic, anti-inflammatory, urinary antiseptic, mild diuretic.

MEDICINAL USE: A classic remedy for nosebleeds and internal bleeding to excessive menstrual loss. Useful in urinary infections and kidney stones.

PREPARATIONS: Infusions, tincture.

DOSE: 2-8g dried herb equivalent three times daily.

Capsicum minimum

(Solanaceae) also *C. frutescens*

CAYENNE, CHILLI, BIRD PEPPER, AFRICAN CHILLI

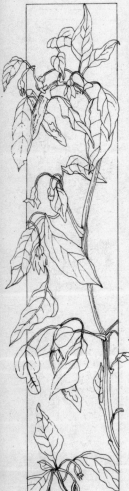

The same hot chilli from Africa and the Caribbean which provides the 'heat' in curries and other spicy foods from Singapore via Madras to Mexico City. Cayenne pepper and Tabasco are kitchen forms. Chillies were recorded by Columbus's doctor on his second voyage to the West Indies in 1494. Only later were they taken to India by the Portuguese traders in a reversal of the Far East spice trade. The African chillies are hotter than the larger Indian chillies and are close relatives of the sweet pepper, or capsicum, from which paprika is made. A perennial growing to 2m (6ft.) with elliptical leaves, small white flowers and distinctive red or yellow oblong fruits to 3cm (1.25in.). Grows easily under glass or in sheltered gardens in temperate areas.

PARTS USED: Fruits.

ACTIVE INGREDIENTS/ACTIONS: An alkaloid, capsaicin; carotenoids; saponins known as capsicidins; flavonoids; volatile oil. Central circulatory stimulant, diaphoretic, spasmolytic, antiseptic, rubifacient.

MEDICINAL USE: Used where reduced circulation is a factor, including digestive debility, flatulent colic, reduced peripheral circulation. Used topically to draw in healing blood in joint inflammation, unbroken chilblains, lumbago. Only small doses are used to avoid irritating the stomach or burning the skin.

PREPARATIONS: Tincture, food spice, creams.

DOSE: 0.05–0.5g dried herb equivalent three times daily.

Carduus marianus

(Compositae) also *Silybum marianum*

MILK THISTLE, MARIA THISTLE

Despite the defensive barrier of prickles on the leaves, this and the related holy thistle were a favourite vegetable. Both thistles have a long medical pedigree. Culpeper claimed it 'helps plague-sores, boils and itch, the bitings of mad dogs and venomous beasts'. Gerard and Dioscorides before him used it for liver diseases, an indication that modern medicine has confirmed. One ingredient, known as silimarin, has been shown to protect liver cells from damage from toxins and to stimulate regrowth of damaged liver cells. A native of southern Europe, it is naturalized in the United States and cultivated in many other countries. Thistle-like annual with wavy, toothed leaves which are dark green with distinctive white veins. Cultivated easily from seed.

PARTS USED: Seeds.

ACTIVE INGREDIENTS/ACTIONS: Flavolignans, including silibin, known collectively as silimarin. Liver protective, bitter, antihaemorrhagic.

MEDICINAL USE: Used in dyspepsia or sluggish digestion related to liver function; excellent in viral hepatitis and degenerative liver disease, especially due to toxins like alcohol or drugs.

PREPARATIONS: Infusion, tincture.

DOSE: 1-5g seeds equivalent three times daily.

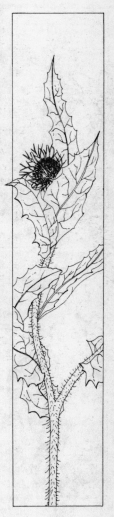

Cassia senna

(Leguminosae) also *C. acutifolia* and *C. angustifolia*

SENNA, ALEXANDRIAN SENNA, NUBIAN SENNA, CASSIA SENNA, TINNEVELLY SENNA

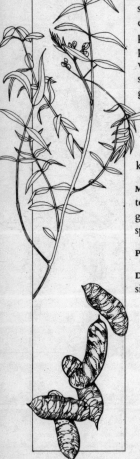

Several East African species supply the main commercial crop. The Arabian physicians who imported material through Alexandria were among the first to record use of senna leaf as medicine. Senna provides the main ingredient of many pharmaceutical laxatives. A small shrubby plant with stems angled upwards. Leaves are in opposite pairs about 1.5cm (0.5in.) long. Small yellow flowers give way to flat, slightly curved 5cm (2in.) pods containing 6 seeds. Cultivation difficult in temperate countries without glasshouse conditions.

PARTS USED: Leaves, pods.

ACTIVE INGREDIENTS/ACTIONS: Anthraquinone glycosides; sennosides A and B; aloe-emodin; rhein; kaempferol; mucilage; calcium oxalate. Stimulant laxative.

MEDICINAL USE: For short-term use in constipation due to lack of tone or peristalsis in the bowel. Combine with ginger, fennel or cardamom to reduce griping. Avoid in spastic constipation or colitis.

PREPARATIONS: Infusion, tablets, tincture.

DOSE: 2–8g dried herb equivalent taken as tablet or infusion before bed.

Caulophyllum thalictroides

(Berberidaceae)

BLUE COHOSH, PAPOOSE ROOT, SQUAW ROOT, BLUE GINSENG

One of the many herbs adopted after studying the Native Americans' use of it to encourage a painless and easy childbirth, hence the common name. It was once included in the United States pharmacopoeia. A native of North America and one of the Indian medicines brought to Europe during the nineteenth century. Found in moist mountain valleys. A tortuous branching rootstock sends up erect stems with pinnate leaves, each of which has leaflets with 2-3 lobes. Small six-petalled flowers appear in early summer at the tip of stems and produce small black seeds.

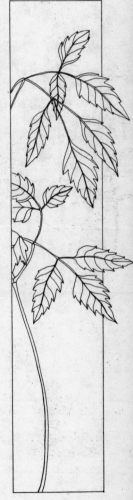

PARTS USED: Root.

ACTIVE INGREDIENTS/ACTIONS: Alkaloids, including caulophylline; steroidal saponin, caulosaponin. Strong expectorant, emmenagogue, spasmolytic, uterine tonic, anti-inflammatory.

MEDICINAL USE: Used mainly for tense uterine conditions including painful periods, functional lack of periods, pains in pelvic inflammation and fibroids. Also used in rheumatism. Avoid in the pregnancy until labour has begun.

PREPARATIONS: Decoction of dried root, tincture.

DOSE: 1-5g dried herb equivalent three times daily.

Centaurium erythraea

(Gentianaceae) also *Erythraea centaurium*

CENTAURY, RED CENTAURY, FILWORT, CHRIST'S LADDER

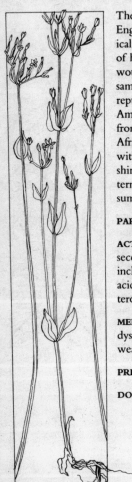

The generic name comes from the Greek for 'red'. The English common name, centaury, derives from the mythical centaur, Chironia, who was a renowned practitioner of herbal medicine and cured one of his poisoned arrow wounds with centaury. It is a classic bitter herb from the same family as gentian (q.v.) and has a long-established reputation as a healer of wounds and infections. The American centaury is a different plant (*Sabbatia angularis*) from the same family. A native of Europe and North Africa. It grows wild in dry alkaline soils. A tufted annual with a square stem rising to 40cm (16in.) with pale green, shiny lanceolate leaves placed opposite without petioles. A terminal cluster of red, five-petalled flowers appears in late summer. Cultivation is difficult.

PARTS USED: Leaves and stem.

ACTIVE INGREDIENTS/ACTIONS: Glycosides known as secoiroids, including sweroside, gentiopicrin; alkaloids including gentianine, gentioflavine; xanthones; phenolic acids; triterpenes including sitosterol, campesterol, stigmasterol. Bitter, stomachic, tonic.

MEDICINAL USE: Used in sluggish digestion, anorexia, dyspepsia, especially where there is liver or gall bladder weakness. Bitters are taken before food.

PREPARATIONS: Infusion, tincture.

DOSE: 1-3g dried herb equivalent three times daily.

Cephaelis ipecacuanha

(Rubiaceae)

IPECACUANHA ROOT, MATTO GROSSO

'Ipec' is one of the romantic herbal medicines discovered and is still harvested from the trees of the tropical forests of Brazil where it is native. A Portuguese friar who lived in Brazil around 1600 learned of its powers from the local natives. In 1670, it became popular in Europe as a treatment for dysentery in the form of a patent medicine manufactured by one Dr Helvetius. A perennial with a fibrous root sending up angular stems to 30cm (12in.) with opposite, oval leaves. Clusters of small mauve flowers appear in the autumn and produce small purple berries. Cultivation difficult.

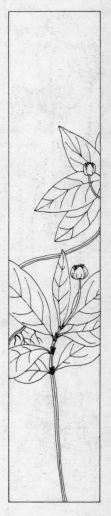

PARTS USED: Roots.

ACTIVE INGREDIENTS/ACTIONS: Alkaloids, especially emetamine, cephaline and protoemetine; tannins; glycosides; saponins. Expectorant, emetic, antiprotozoal.

MEDICINAL USE: A potent expectorant in chronic bronchitis and pertussis; and an emetic in larger doses. Useful in drug overdose where the stomach needs immediate emptying; effective against amoebae in dysentery. Large doses are emetic and irritant to the whole intestine and should be used only under professional supervision.

PREPARATIONS: Decoction, tincture, ingredient in proprietary cough medicines.

DOSE: 0.25-1g dried herb equivalent three times daily as expectorant. 1-5g as an emetic.

Cetaria icelandica

(Parmeliaceae)

ICELAND MOSS, CETARIA

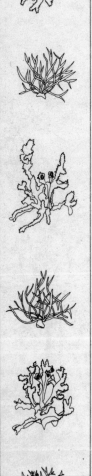

This is not a moss but a lichen, which is a mutually bene-ficial combination of an alga and a fungus. Its habitat is dry, stony, barren ground in the higher latitudes – north-ern Europe, Iceland, the North American tundra and even in Antarctica. It contains up to 70 per cent 'lichen starch' and has long been used as emergency food of humans and wild animals in desolate places. The plant body, or thallus, is perennial, erect, much branched and curly to 10cm (4in.) high. It is grey-brown or olive on top and paler with tiny white spots underneath. Cannot be cultivated.

PARTS USED: Thallus.

ACTIVE INGREDIENTS/ACTIONS
Mucilaginous polysaccharides, especially lichenin and iso-lichenin; bitter acids including fumarprotocetraric, cetraric, lichesteric, usnic. Demulcent, expectorant, anti-emetic, antibiotic.

MEDICINAL USE: In gastritis, dyspepsia with vomiting, res-piratory catarrh and bronchitis.

PREPARATIONS: Decoction, cold infusion, tincture. It is a common ingredient of proprietary cough medicines.

DOSE: 5–10g dried herb equivalent three times daily.

Chamaelerium luteum

(Liliaceae)

HELONIAS, FALSE UNICORN ROOT, STARWORT

Another of the many herbs learned of from the Native Americans' detailed knowledge of herbs for the female reproductive system. A perennial growing in wet, marshy places in the south-east of the United States, growing to 1m (3ft.) with lanceolate leaves 15–20cm (6–8in.) long and producing a terminal plume of small green-white flowers, with separate male and female forms, in late summer. There is a small, round rhizome about 3cm (1in.) in diameter.

PARTS USED: Rhizome.

ACTIVE INGREDIENTS/ACTIONS: Saponins; glycosides including chamaelirin and helonin. Uterine tonic, diuretic, anthelmintic.

MEDICINAL USE: For absent or painful periods, threatened miscarriage, nausea in pregnancy, and in female infertility due to ovarian malfunction.

PREPARATIONS: Infusion, tincture.

DOSE: 4–10g dried herb equivalent three times daily.

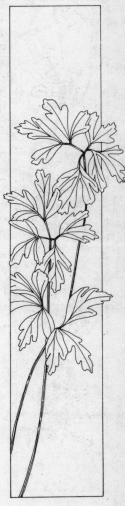

Chelidonium majus

(Papaveraceae)

GREATER CELANDINE, COMMON CELANDINE

The Greek philosopher, Pliny the Great, knew this herb. It is included in nearly all of the famous herbals. It is said to be named after the Greek for 'swallows' because it starts flowering when they arrive and stops when they leave. But Aristotle has a more imaginative explanation. He claimed it was so named because it restores the eyes of swallows 'if a man do prick them out'. Native to Europe but introduced throughout the temperate world. A perennial with small stems growing to 60cm (2ft.) with deeply cut leaves which are pale green, thin and hairy. The stem oozes a rich orange latex if cut or broken. Small clusters of bright yellow, delicate flowers are produced all summer and they give way to thin pods 3–5cm (1–2in.). Readily cultivated from seed or root division.

PARTS USED: Whole herb during flowering.

ACTIVE INGREDIENTS/ACTIONS: Alkaloids including berberine, chelamine, chelidonine; saponins; choline. Spasmolytic, bitter, cholagogue, laxative and diuretic.

MEDICINAL USE: For jaundice; gall stones and gall bladder disease, especially inflammation; topically for eczema, verrucae and other warts. Has been used to reduce cataracts. Should be used only under professional supervision.

PREPARATIONS: Infusion, tincture.

DOSE: 1–3g dried herb equivalent three times daily.

Cimicifuga racemosa

(Ranunculaceae)

BLACK COHOSH, BLACK SNAKE ROOT, RATTLE ROOT, SQUAW ROOT

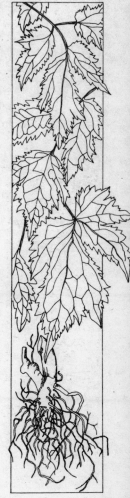

Along with many other herbs throughout history, this was claimed to cure the poisonous bites of snakes, in this case the rattlesnakes of North America. The Native Americans used it also to ease the pain of menstruation and birth for their squaws. The early settlers brought the herb back to European medicine in the nineteenth century. A native to North America and grows in open woodland. A perennial growing to 1.25m (4.1ft.) with a smooth stem carrying compound leaves having ovate leaflets with serrated margins. The flowers are in a spike of strong smelling, creamy-white flowers produced in summer. The root and rhizome are black. Not easily cultivated.

PARTS USED: Root and rhizome collected in autumn.

ACTIVE INGREDIENTS/ACTIONS: Triterpene glycosides including actein, cimifugine and racemoside; isoflavones; ranunculin which converts to anemonin. Antispasmodic, anti-inflammatory, alterative, sedative, vasodilator.

MEDICINAL USE: Used in painful period spasms and in leucorrhoea; in inflammatory conditions with cramps or pain; in muscular rheumatism, neuralgia, muscle cramps, myalgia; in paroxysmal coughing in bronchitis or whooping cough.
Warning: This herb should be used only under professional supervision and should not be used in pregnancy.

PREPARATIONS: Decoction, tincture.

DOSE: 0.5-1 dried rhizome equivalent three times daily.

Commiphora molmol

(Burseraceae)

MYRRH, MYRRHA, MIRRA, DIDTHIN

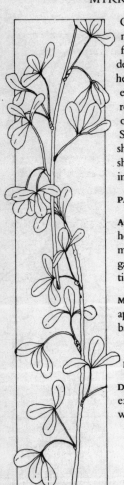

One of the precious gifts to the infant Christ and widely mentioned elsewhere in the Bible. It was used as a perfume in ancient Egyptian embalming fluids. Its name may derive from the Greek legend of Myrrh. The gods turned her into a tree to hide her from her father's rage at discovering he had been tricked into incest. The exudates of resin from the cut bark are said to be her tears. A native of the driest parts of north-east Africa and Arabia, but Somalia was and remains the principal source of drug. The shrub grows to 3m (9ft.) with gnarled branches and many short sub-branches that carry small trifoliate leaves and end in a tough spine. Cultivation difficult.

PARTS USED: Resin.

ACTIVE INGREDIENTS/ACTIONS: Volatile oil containing heerabolene, canidene, eugenol; resins including commiphoric acids, commiphorinic acid; gums of arabinose, galactose, xylose; sterols. Stimulant, expectorant, antiseptic, anti–inflammatory, vulnerary.

MEDICINAL USE: Extremely effective in mouthwashes for aphthous ulcers, inflamed gums, and sore throats. Helps in bacterial lung infections and catarrhal congestion. Used topically for wounds and abrasions.

PREPARATIONS: Tincture, tablets.

DOSE: 0.5-1g dried resin equivalent three times daily as expectorant, but larger amounts as tincture for mouthwashes or wound lotions.

Convallaria majalis

(Liliaceae)

LILY–OF–THE–VALLEY, MAY LILY, MUGET

Ancient healers long recognized the value of this herb in 'disorders of the heart and vital spirits', without realizing its valuable action on the heart and hence the circulation in the brain. It has greater safety than the other important heart herb, the foxglove (*Digitalis* spp.) from which the active ingredients, digoxin and digitoxin, have been extracted and turned into a pharmaceutical medicine. A native of Europe, North America and northern Asia, where it grows in the drier parts of shady woods. An underground stem sends up two ovate leaves without petioles to about 20cm (8in.). In spring, the characteristic bell-shaped white flowers are borne on an erect spike. The fragrance is strong and pleasant. Easily cultivated.

PARTS USED: Leaves during flowering.

ACTIVE INGREDIENTS/ACTIONS: Glycosides convallatoxin, convalloside, convallatoxol; flavonoids; asparagin. Cardioactive, diuretic.

MEDICINAL USE: Used in congestive heart failure where it releases its active glycosides more slowly than *Digitalis* and is thus less likely to cause a toxic build-up. To relieve the oedema of cardiac failure. **Warning:** Not to be taken except on a herbalist's supervision.

PREPARATIONS: Tincture.

DOSE: 0.15g dried herb equivalent three times daily.

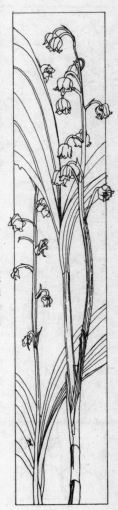

Crateagus oxycanthus

(Rosaceae) also *C. monogyna*

MAY, WHITETHORN, HAW, BREAD AND CHEESE

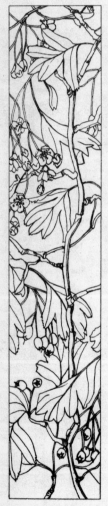

Hawthorn flowers in May stand out in hedgerows or woods. They are reputed to have magical properties and it is still considered bad luck to take them into homes. It was chosen as a symbol by Henry VII and is said to have been source of Christ's crown of thorns. The generic name comes from the Greek for strong and refers to the hard wood. The specific name, *oxycanthus*, derives from two words meaning sharp thorn. Native to Europe, North Africa and West Asia and introduced to other temperate countries. This shrub or small tree grows to 10m (33ft.) with deeply lobed, dark-green leaves, and clusters of white flowers from early to midsummer. Trees are laden with oval red berries in the autumn. Readily cultivated.

PARTS USED: Flowers, leaves, fruits.

ACTIVE INGREDIENTS/ACTIONS: Flavonoids, including quercetin, rutin, vitexin; cyano-genic glycosides including procyanidine; phenolic acids, including chlorogenic; tannins; ascorbic acid. Coronary and peripheral vasodilator; cardiac tonic; hypotensive; relieves tachycardia.

MEDICINAL USE: A valuable heart tonic. It improves coronary blood flow and efficiency in heart failure; helps peripheral circulation and intermittent claudication in atherosclerosis; relieves angina pain; lowers high and raises low blood pressure. **Warning:** Never treat heart conditions without professional advice.

PREPARATIONS: Infusion, tincture.

DOSE: 2–10g dried herb equivalent three times daily.

Datura stramonium

(Solanaceae)

JIMSON WEED, THORN APPLE, DEVIL'S APPLE, JAMESTOWN WEED

A toxic plant that must be treated with respect as its common name, devil's apple, warns. The American names, Jimson and Jamestown weed, were earned when, in 1676, a garrison of troops were disabled for several days by its effects which include double vision, urine retention and hallucinations. A native to both western Asia around the Caspian Sea and to the Americas, where it is found on open waste ground. It was introduced to Europe as a drug in the sixteenth century. Gerard recommended a salve made from the leaves boiled in 'hogs grease' for 'all inflammations whatsoever, [including] boiling lead, gunpowder [*sic*], as that which comes by lightning'. A strong-smelling annual to 1.5m (5ft.) with large, soft, ovate leaves up to 20cm (8in.) long. Funnel-shaped blue to white flowers appear in late summer and are followed by an egg-shaped capsule covered in spines, which opens by splitting into four segments displaying the brown seeds. Easily cultivated.

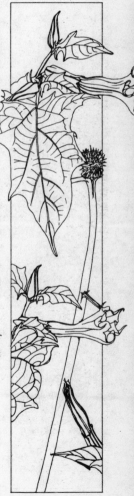

PARTS USED: Leaves, seeds.

ACTIVE INGREDIENTS/ACTIONS: Tropane alkaloids, including hyoscamine, hyoscine, atropine. Spasmolytic, antiasthmatic, anticholinergic.

MEDICINAL USE: For asthma and the muscle spasm of Parkinson's disease. **Warning:** Poisonous and should not be taken except under professional supervision.

PREPARATIONS: Infusions, tincture, leaf tobacco.

DOSE: 0.05g dried herb equivalent three times daily.

Digitalis purpurea

(Scrophulariaceae) also related species *D. lanata*

FOXGLOVE, WITCHES' GLOVES, BLOODY FINGERS, VIRGIN'S GLOVE, FAIRY CAPS

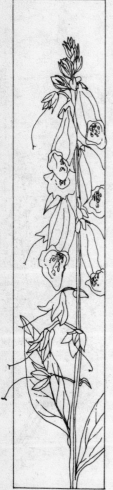

A traditional inclusion in remedies for dropsy (fluid retention). Only when an English doctor, William Withering, identified it as the active herb in one English folk recipe for dropsy, was its value in heart disease accepted. Heart failure is one common cause of dropsy, which is swelling caused by the accumulation of body fluids. The pharmaceutical industry extracts the plant's alkaloids to make the drug digoxin. A biennial with a rosette of thick, down-covered ovate leaves out of which rises a single spike of mauve to purple trumpet flowers in midsummer. Native to western Europe but cultivated in gardens around the world. Prefers light acid soils.

PARTS USED: Leaves.

ACTIVE INGREDIENTS/ACTIONS: Cardioactive glycosides, including digitoxin, gitoxin. *D. lanata* also contains digoxin. Increased heartbeat efficiency (inotrophic), diuretic.

MEDICINAL USE: In congestive heart failure. The leaf has been shown to be less toxic than the extracted drug, and requires smaller doses. **Warning:** The plant is poisonous and should not be taken except under professional advice.

PREPARATIONS: Leaf extract.

DOSE: 0.1mg digoxin equivalent twice daily.

Dioscorea villosa

(Dioscoriaceae)

WILD YAM, COLIC ROOT, RHEUMATISM ROOT, DIOSCOREA

Yams are underground storage stems and a popular food crop throughout the tropics. A related species, *D. mexicana*, was the original source of synthetic hormones for the manufacture of the female contraceptive pill. Wild yam was used as a resource until 1970. In China, three *Dioscorea* species are used to extract drugs. A native of eastern and central United States. It is perennial, with long and twisted roots and a twinning stem with small heart-shaped leaves and green to yellow flowers in drooping panicles in the summer. Easily cultivated but takes 3-5 years to produce yams.

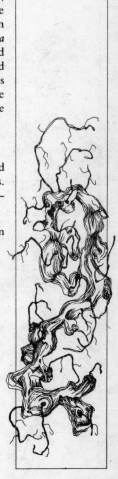

PARTS USED: Root or rhizome.

ACTIVE INGREDIENTS/ACTIONS: Steroidal saponins based on diosgenin including dioscin, dioscorin; starch; tannins. Spasmolytic, peripheral vasodilator, cholagogue, anti-inflammatory.

MEDICINAL USE: For inflamed joints or muscles in rheumatic disease; spasm or inflammation in the gut; in diverticulitis; cramps and intermittent claudication; painful periods; ovarian and uterine pain.

PREPARATIONS: Decoction, tincture.

DOSE: 2-5g dried herb equivalent three times daily.

Echinacea angustifolia

(Compositae)

CONEFLOWER, PURPLE CONEFLOWER, BLACK SAMPSON, KANSAS SNAKEROOT

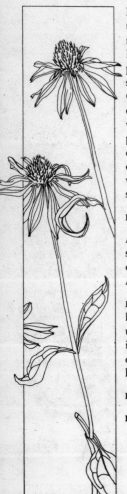

Echinacea has been known to increase resistance to infection for centuries. Science has shown that it increases the number of white blood cells that fight infection. Both Native Americans and the early settlers used this plant for protecting wounds from infections, and even to cure snakebites. It is also antiviral and is being studied in California as a possible treatment for AIDS. A native of central and south-western United States but domesticated varieties are widely grown in gardens across the world. It prefers dry open ground. Perennial to 1m (3ft.) with coarse hairy stems and sparse lanceolate leaves also with coarse hairs. Terminal flowers have a raised cone of florets with an outer ring of purple-ray florets and appear in late summer. Easily cultivated.

PARTS USED: Roots and rhizome.

ACTIVE INGREDIENTS/ACTIONS: Glycoside, echinacoside; echinacin; polysaccharides; polyacetylenes; essential oil, including humulene; caryophyllene; flavonoids. Antiseptic, antiviral, immune stimulant, alterative.

MEDICINAL USE: To disinfect wounds and encourage healing, especially in boils, carbuncles and septicaemia; useful in upper respiratory tract infections, including influenza, tonsillitis and pharyngitis. Sipped regularly it combats flu infections. As an alterative in skin conditions like eczema and psoriasis.

PREPARATIONS: Decoction, tincture, tablets.

DOSE: 2–10ml dried herb equivalent three times daily.

Elutherococcus senticosus

(Araliaceae)

SIBERIAN GINSENG, TAIGA ROOT

Not to be confused with the Asiatic ginseng (*Panax ginseng*), which is the herb usually referred to by the common name, 'ginseng'. Russian workers have found significant increases in the stamina of trained athletes and astronauts treated with the herb. It is known as an adaptogen, which means it increases the resistance of the body to adverse conditions. A native of Siberia, the Himalayan area and south-east Asia. It is a prickly shrub that grows to 6m (20ft.). The palmate leaves have red petioles and up to 5 elliptical, serrated leaflets. Small umbels of white flowers appear at the tips of stems, resolving into small round fruits. Can be cultivated with care.

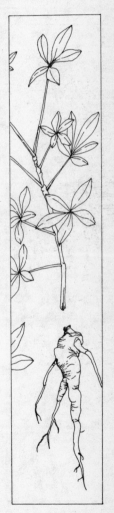

PARTS USED: Roots.

ACTIVE INGREDIENTS/ACTIONS: Glycosides known as eleutherosides, known as A, B, B_1, C, D, E, and F; sugars; volatile oils; Vitamins C, E; Chlorogenic acid; and minerals. Adaptogen, which includes immunostimulation, increases stress tolerance, reduces effects of toxins in the body, antiviral, antihypertensive.

PREPARATIONS: Tincture, tablets.

DOSE: 1–15g dried herb equivalent three times daily.

Ephedra sinica

(Ephedraceae)

EPHEDRA, MA HUANG

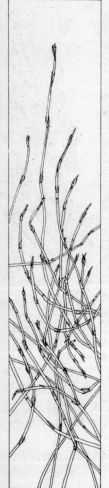

One of many Chinese herbs that have found an important place in Western medicine. *Ephedra* has been used for asthma in Chinese medicine for 5,000 years. The ingredient ephedrine was isolated in 1887 and became an effective pharmaceutical drug for use in asthma. Because of the way it helps asthma, it can also raise blood pressure. However, the whole plant is safer as it contains other ingredients which help lower blood pressure even while easing the asthma. A living fossil plant which is native to the Himalayas and the mountains of China. A short shrub with smooth, green and grooved branches with leaves reduced to tufts. Separate male and female flowers are produced in summer followed by small succulent cones.

PARTS USED: Young stems.

ACTIVE INGREDIENTS/ACTIONS: Alkaloids including ephedrine, pseudoephedrine, norephedrine. Anti-asthmatic, bronchodilator, cardiac stimulant, peripheral vasoconstrictor.

MEDICINAL USE: Specific for bronchial asthma where it eases the severity and frequency of bronchial spasms; for urticaria and other allergies. **Warning:** The drug should be used only under professional supervision and avoided in cases of high blood pressure, glaucoma, and hyperthyroidism or in patients taking MAOI drugs.

PREPARATIONS: Infusion, tincture.

DOSE: 0.05–0.6g dried herb equivalent three times daily.

Equisetum arvense

(Equisetaceae)

HORSETAIL, BOTTLEBRUSH, SHAVE GRASS, DUTCH RUSHES

The horsetails are common finds among fossils from the carboniferous period. It has been used since ancient Greek and Roman times as a vegetable, animal feed, scourer for pewter ware, and medicine. Culpeper said it was 'very powerful to stop bleeding either inward or outward ... and eases the swelling heat and inflammation of the fundamental, or privy parts, in men and women.' A robust perennial native to Europe and found on damp or heavy clay soils, where its presence indicates ground water. Two types of stems rise from a wandering rhizome. Fertile stems appear in early spring, and are followed by vegetative stems to 50cm (19in.). The latter are jointed and have toothed sheaths, instead of leaves, arising from the joints like spokes of a wheel. Cultivation easy, but it spreads voraciously.

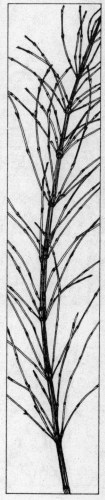

PARTS USED: Vegetative stems.

ACTIVE INGREDIENTS/ACTIONS: Alkaloids including nicotine, palustrine and palustrinine; saponins; flavonoids including isoquercetin, equicetrin; sterols, including cholesterol; silicic acid; minerals. Haemostatic, astringent, styptic, stimulates immune response.

MEDICINAL USE: An astringent in urinary and prostate diseases to stop bleeding, relieve inflammation and aid healing; used in juvenile bedwetting; as a healer in lung disease.

PREPARATIONS: Infusion, decoction, tincture.

DOSE: 2–8g dried herb equivalent three times daily.

Eucalyptus globulus

(Myrtaceae) and related species

BLUE GUM, TASMANIAN BLUE GUM, GUM TREE, EUCALYPT

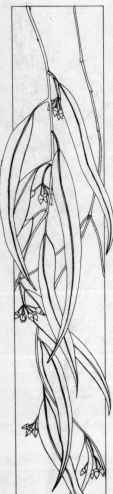

Eucalypts, or gum trees, are almost a trademark of the Australian landscape. Out of 300 species of Eucalypts, 30 have found medicinal use. The aborigines were using the leaves for chest infections 40,000 years ago. An early white Australian immigrant, Joseph Bosito, first extracted the volatile oils in 1848 by distilling them out with steam. The plant is effective at draining swamps and has been used in malaria mosquito eradication programmes in Africa, Southern Europe and India. Crushed leaves have been used as a household insect repellent. Native to Australia but now grown in North Africa, Spain, Portugal and California. The trees grow to 115m (375ft.) with a smooth bluish-grey trunk and long narrow leathery leaves with a bluish-green hue and many oil glands. Flowering is during late summer. Fruits are shaped like spinning tops with a coating of powdery wax. Cultivation easy.

PARTS USED: Leaves.

ACTIVE INGREDIENTS/ACTIONS: Volatile oil mainly 1,8-cineole or eucalyptol, with terpineole, pinene; polyphenolic acids including caffeic, gallic; flavonoids including eucalyptin, hyperoside and rutin. Antiseptic, antispasmodic, expectorant, stimulant, febrifuge.

MEDICINAL USE: A common ingredient of cough medicines; as vapour rub for colds or other respiratory infections; or as a rubifacient for bruised or strained muscles. Widely used in pharmaceutical products and in the flavouring and cosmetic industries.

PREPARATIONS: Essential oil, tincture.

DOSE: 0.05–0.1ml dried herb equivalent three times daily.

Eupatorium perfoliatum

(Compositae)

BONESET, FEVERWORT, THOROUGHWORT

The first white settlers of North America relied on this Native American herb to tackle a serious flu-like disease called 'break bone fever'. The local name was 'ague weed'. Native to the east coast of North America in marshy soils. It is a perennial growing to 1m (39in.) with lanceolate leaves in opposite pairs, each leaf closely joined to the stem. Flowers appear in late summer as a cluster of densely packed, small white or bluish flowers at the top of stems. Cultivation is possible with care.

PARTS USED: Whole herb.

ACTIVE INGREDIENTS/ACTIONS: Volatile oils including sesquiterpene lactones; glycoside, eupatorin; polysaccharides; flavonoids including quercetin, kaempferol, rutin. Diaphoretic and peripheral vasodilator, cholagogue, antispasmodic, gentle laxative.

MEDICINAL USE: Specific for influenza; used in bronchitis and in chronic nasal catarrh; used in rheumatoid arthritis made worse by damp.

PREPARATIONS: Infusion, tincture.

DOSE: 0.5–4g dried herb equivalent three times daily.

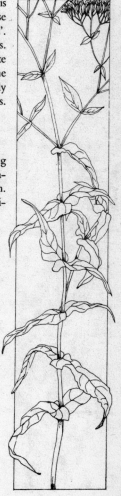

Euphrasia officinalis

(Scrophulariaceae)

EYEBRIGHT, MEADOW EYEBRIGHT, CASSE LUNETTE
AUGENTRÖST

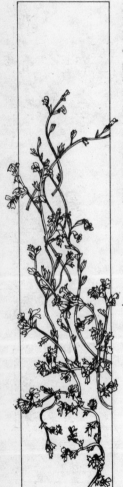

Named after Euphrosne, one of the three Greek graces. First used as a medicine by the abbess and herbalist, Hildegarde, in the twelfth century to 'strengthen the head, eyes, and memory'. A native of Europe's well-drained, grassy meadows and hills, but also found in western Asia and North America. A semi-parasitic plant always found in association with meadow grass host. An erect annual growing to 30cm (12in.) with opposite, oval and toothed leaves. The flower has a double-lobed lower lip and a toothed calyx with glandular hairs. The lower lip has a yellow patch and fine red or purple veins resembling a bloodshot eye. Flowering is from mid to late summer. Cultivation difficult.

PARTS USED: Herb during flowering.

ACTIVE INGREDIENTS/ACTIONS: Glycosides, including acubin; tannins; phenolic acids; volatile oils; choline. Anti-catarrhal, astringent, anti-inflammatory.

MEDICINAL USE: As a mucosal membrane toner in nasal and upper respiratory catarrh, and sinusitis; useful in conjunctivitis.

PREPARATIONS: Infusion, tincture.

DOSE: 2–8g dried herb equivalent three times daily.

Fagopyrum esculentum

(Polygonaceae)

BUCKWHEAT, BLE NOIR, SARACEN CORN, BUCHWEIZEN

Buckwheat is not a grass and is no relation of wheat (*Tritiaum* spp.). It is native of Central Asia and China where it is used as a flour. In Europe and North America it is made into flour for making cakes and crumpets, which are griddle toasted in Holland. An annual with erect stems bearing arrow-shaped, soft leaves, and topped by panicles of small pinkish flowers in summer. The seeds are small three-sided pyramids. Cultivation easy.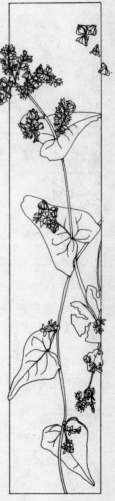

PARTS USED: Leaves.

ACTIVE INGREDIENTS/ACTIONS: Flavonoid glycosides rutin and quercetin. Antihaemorrhagic, vasodilator, and repairing to blood vessel walls.

MEDICINAL USE: For any causes of capillary fragility; in varicose veins; in frostbite and chilblains, retinal haemorrhages, and radiation damage.

PREPARATIONS: Infusion, tablets.

DOSE: 2–10g dried herb equivalent, three times daily.

Filipendula ulmaria

also *Spiraea ulmaria (Rosaceae)*

MEADOWSWEET, QUEEN OF THE MEADOW, BRIDEWORT, DOLLOFF

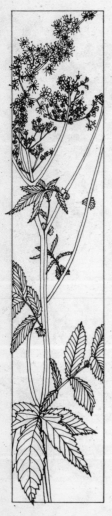

Meadowsweet was the plant in which a German chemist first identified methyl salicylate, which was later synthesized in a slightly changed form as aspirin. It also used to be a flavouring for mead and was known as 'meadwort'. Unlike aspirin, which can cause stomach inflammation, meadowsweet is safer and is used to treat stomach inflammations like gastritis. Native to Europe and Asia but now naturalized in North America. A perennial with erect, brittle, reddish stems to 120cm (47in.) bearing alternate pairs of pinnate leaves with tough, serrated leaflets. The exquisitely sweet-scented flowers appear in mid to late summer as clusters of tiny white or cream cymes at the top of stems. Easily cultivated.

PARTS USED: Herb harvested during flowering.

ACTIVE INGREDIENTS/ACTIONS: Salicylic glycosides including spiraein and gaultherin; flavonoids including rutin, spiraeoside, and hyperoside; tannins; coumarin; ascorbic acid. Stomachic, antirheumatic, antacid, anti-inflammatory, astringent, diaphoretic, mild urinary antiseptic.

MEDICINAL USE: A gentle and safe healer in peptic ulcer and other stomach inflammation; dyspepsia with heartburn; rheumatic pain of joints and muscles; helps with diarrhoea in children.

PREPARATIONS: Infusion, tincture.

DOSE: 2–8g dried herb equivalent three times daily.

Foeniculum vulgare

(Umbelliferae)

FENNEL, SWEET FENNEL, FENKEL

A highly respected food and medicine for centuries. It was once thought to be good for eyesight after watching snakes rub their heads on the plant after shedding skin. Pliny used it for more than 20 ailments, including improving eyesight and as a carminative to 'break the wind'. Native to southern Europe, it is now naturalized all over the world and widely cultivated for food and medicine. A hardy perennial with a blue-green, ribbed stem to 2m (6.5ft.) bearing feathery leaves with broad, wrap-around petioles. A dense collection of yellow flowers in umbels appears in mid–late summer, followed by greyish oblong fruit with a taste of anise. Cultivation easy.

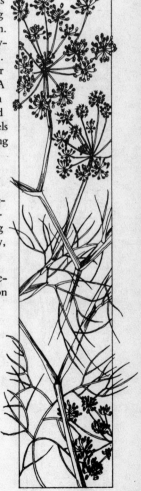

PARTS USED: Fruit.

ACTIVE INGREDIENTS/ACTIONS: Volatile oil with anethole, fenchone, limonene and apiole; flavonoids including rutin, kaempferol and quercetin; coumarins including bergapten. Stomachic, carminative, anti-inflammatory, orexigenic, galactagogue.

MEDICINAL USE: For flatulent dyspepsia and colic, especially in children; and useful stimulant of milk production in breast-feeding.

PREPARATIONS: Infusion, dried fruits, tincture.

DOSE: 2-12g dried herb equivalent three times daily.

Galium aparine

(Rubiaceae)

CLEAVERS, CLIVERS, GOOSE GRASS, CATCH GRASS, MUTTON CHOPS, HAYRIFFE, ERRIFFE

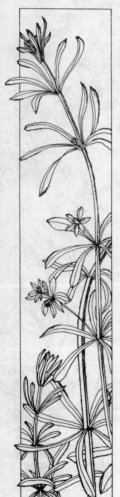

The coffee tree is a close relative and the seeds of cleavers make a passable coffee substitute. A centuries-old treatment for skin diseases and purifying the blood. When combined with nettle tops, it makes the once popular 'spring cleansing' tonic for the liver and blood. Culpeper said it is a good remedy 'to cleanse the blood and strengthen the liver, thereby to keep the body in health, and fitting it for that change of season that is coming'. A native of Europe in damp semi-shaded land but widely spread through temperate world. It is a distinctive annual with trailing habit. Quadrangular stems carry narrow, lance-shaped leaves in whorls of 6 or 8 around the stem. Both leaves and stems are covered in fine hooks which help the plant cling to other plants it climbs over or anything it touches. Easily cultivated.

PARTS USED: Whole herb.

ACTIVE INGREDIENTS/ACTIONS: Coumarins; iridoids, flavonoids; tannins. Diuretic, astringent, lymphatic alterative.

MEDICINAL USE: Helpful in skin rashes of the eczema type; in swollen lymph glands especially with oedema and water retention; helpful in urinary infections and stones.

PREPARATIONS: Infusions, tincture.

DOSE: 2–10g dried herb equivalent three times daily.

Gaultheria procumbens

(Ericaceae)

WINTERGREEN, TEABERRY, CHECKERBERRY

The leaves of this small herb have been used as an aromatic tea and an animal feed. It is a commercial source of natural methyl salicylates, which are anti-inflammatory and found in the distilled oil. Most oil of wintergreen now sold is either synthetic or derived from a birch tree (*Betula* spp.). A native of North America, this small perennial shrubby plant grows to 15cm (6in.), with stiff erect branches bearing tufts of oval leaves at their apex. Drooping white flowers appear from the base of leaves in midsummer and develop into red berries. It thrives on poor, dry and sandy soils.

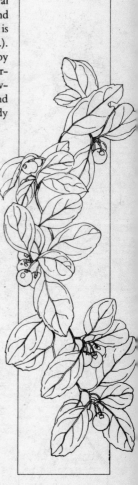

PARTS USED: Leaves.

ACTIVE INGREDIENTS/ACTIONS: Phenolic compounds including salicylic acid, gaultherin, vanillic and caffeic acids; volatile oil with methyl salicylate. Anti-inflammatory, diuretic, antirheumatic.

MEDICINAL USE: For relief of painful muscles and joints in rheumatoid arthritis and rheumatism; in myalgia, sprains, and sciatica.

PREPARATIONS: Liniments, ointments.

DOSE: 0.1–2g dried herb equivalent three times daily.

Gelsemium sempervirens

(Loganiaceae)

YELLOW JASMINE ROOT, FALSE JASMINE, WILD WOODBINE, CAROLINA JASMINE

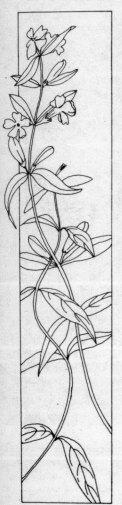

Not related to the scented European jasmines. Originally used for fevers by the early American settlers but is now used only for facial neuralgia and other nerve pain. A native of North America, where it is found around damp lowland soils near water. A perennial climber with opposite, green, lanceolate leaves bearing fragrant clusters of one to five trumpet-shaped yellow flowers in the axils. Flowering is early spring. Easily cultivated.

PARTS USED: Roots and rhizome.

ACTIVE INGREDIENTS/ACTIONS: Alkaloids including gelsemine, gelsemedine, gelsedine; iridoids; coumarins; tannins. Sedative, analgesic, diaphoretic, antispasmodic.

MEDICINAL USE: Used topically for facial neuralgia or toothache. Its sale is regulated in the UK and other countries. **Warning:** Poisonous. Should be used only by qualified practitioners.

PREPARATIONS: Tincture.

DOSE: 0.025g dried herb equivalent three times daily.

Gentiana lutea

(Gentianaceae)

GENTIAN, YELLOW GENTIAN

A medicine in wide use throughout the world since the time of the ancient Greeks. The generic name is said to derive from Gentius, King of Illyria, who discovered its uses to neutralize poisons. Gentian has a distinct bitter taste. It is used as a reference for bitterness. There are easily 200 related species. This one is a native to Europe and Asia Minor but is distributed widely. An alpine plant found around 1,200m (4,000ft.). The root, which may be 30cm (12in.) long and is thick, throws up an erect stem to 1m (3ft.) with short, opposite, stalkless leaves with a yellowish hue. Flowers appear in spring in the axils of the uppermost few pairs of leaves. Easily cultivated.

PARTS USED: Dried root.

ACTIVE INGREDIENTS/ACTIONS: Bitter glycosides including gentiopicrin, amaropicrin, amaroswerin; xanthones such as gentisein and gentisin; alkaloids including gentianine; phenolic acids. Strong bitter stimulant, digestive stimulant, anti–inflammatory.

MEDICINAL USE: For digestive atony and especially useful in anorexia, digestive inflammations, and in liver and gall bladder disease.

PREPARATIONS: Infusion, tincture, tablets.

DOSE: 0.5–3g dried herb equivalent three times daily.

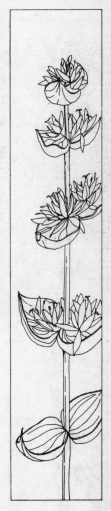

Geranium maculatum

(Gerianaceae)

AMERICAN CRANESBILL, WILD GERANIUM, ALUMROOT, STORKSBILL

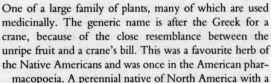

One of a large family of plants, many of which are used medicinally. The generic name is after the Greek for a crane, because of the close resemblance between the unripe fruit and a crane's bill. This was a favourite herb of the Native Americans and was once in the American pharmacopoeia. A perennial native of North America with a hairy stem to 60cm (24in.). Some leaves arise directly from the root but others are opposite on the stem. All leaves are three or four-lobed, hairy, pale green and becoming spotted with age. Rose-pink flowers appear at the apex in late summer. Easily cultivated.

PARTS USED: Rhizome.

ACTIVE INGREDIENTS/ACTIONS: Tannins, including gallic acid. Astringent, styptic, vulnerary, tonic.

MEDICINAL USE: For diarrhoea, intestinal inflammations in enteritis, peptic ulcers, piles and bowel disease. An excellent mouthwash in mouth infections and ulcers, and as a douche in vaginal infections and leucorrhoea.

PREPARATIONS: Infusion, tincture, tablets

DOSE: 1–5g dried herb equivalent three times daily.

Glechoma hederacea

also *Nepeta hederacea (Labitae)*

GROUND IVY, ALEHOOF, LIZZY–RUN–UP–THE–HEDGE, CAT'S FOOT

This is unrelated to true ivies, but the leaves bear a close resemblance. Ground ivy was one of the herbs used to clear ale and flavour it before hops (q.v.) became popular. A traditional cure for coughs and consumption. Native to Europe but naturalized in North America and widely found in temperate regions. A common plant on waste ground and by hedgerows and banks. A low growing perennial with square stems and dark-green heart-shaped leaves with deeply crenated margins. Leaves have a pungent odour. Groups of two or three purple-pink flowers appear in the axils of terminal leaves in spring and summer. Easily cultivated.

PARTS USED: Herb.

ACTIVE INGREDIENTS/ACTIONS: Sesquiterpenes; flavonoids including quercetin, hyperoside, apigenin; saponins; bitter principle, glechomine. Astringent, anticatarrhal, vulnerary, diuretic.

MEDICINAL USE: Used in chronic upper respiratory catarrh, and bronchitis; useful in tinnitus and catarrhal ears; helps reduce symptoms in mild diarrhoea, haemorrhoids and gastritis; relieves cystitis.

PREPARATIONS: Infusions, tincture.

DOSE: 2–8g dried herb equivalent three times daily.

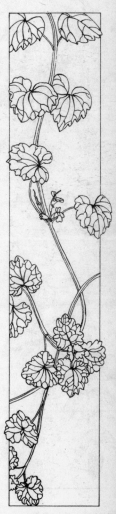

Glycyrrhiza glabra

(Leguminosae)

LIQUORICE, REGLISSE, LACRISSE

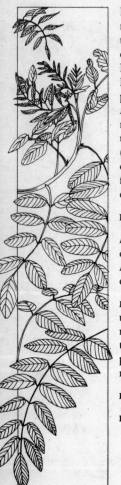

Probably one of the best known and most widely used medicines ever. Its use is recorded from the Assyrian tablets to the 4,000-year-old Chinese herbals. Commercial supplies come from several species with European, Russian, Iranian and Iraqi sources dominating the market. Liquorice extracts are used as a general flavouring for pharmaceutical drugs and foods. Native to Europe and Asia, it is widely grown around the world. It prefers light moist soils along streams. A complex of thick roots sends up erect stems on this perennial which grows to 1.5m (5ft.). Each stem bears up to 7 compound leaves with ovate leaflets, and small pink to violet globular clusters of flowers in the leaf axils during mid to late summer. Easily cultivated.

PARTS USED: Root.

ACTIVE INGREDIENTS/ACTIONS: Glycyrrhizin; glycyrrhetinic acid; flavonoids and isoflavonoids; coumarins. Adrenal cortex stimulant, demulcent, anti-inflammatory, expectorant, spasmolytic, oestrogenic, antiallergic.

MEDICINAL USE: Renowned treatment for peptic ulcer; used in bronchial catarrh, sore throats, gastritis, and in rheumatic conditions; a liver protectant. **Warning:** Long-term usage at high doses may cause sodium retention, low potassium and raised blood pressure, which should be monitored.

PREPARATIONS: Powdered extract, tincture, tablets.

DOSE: 2–8g dried herb equivalent three times daily.

Hamamelis virginica

(Hamamelidaceae)

WITCH–HAZEL, SPOTTED ALDER, WINTERBLOOM

One of the valuable herbs discovered in North America. It was first noticed being used by the Native Americans as a water divining stick and a medicine for skin tumours and related swellings. Now it is widely used in commercial preparations, especially as 'distilled water of witch-hazel' for minor skin irritations and burns. Native to North America. A perennial shrub to 2.5m (8ft.) with smooth bark and ovate leaves with a rough surface and crenated margins. Yellow flowers appear very late in summer to be followed by small black nuts containing white seeds. Cultivation is easy.

PARTS USED: Leaves, bark.

ACTIVE INGREDIENTS/ACTIONS: Tannins; flavonoids including quercetin, kaempferol; saponins. Astringent, anti-haemorrhagic, anti–inflammatory.

MEDICINAL USE: Excellent for haemorrhoids. Useful in diarrhoea, colitis, and locally on inflamed swellings, scalds, and bruises.

PREPARATIONS: Distilled extract, tincture, ointments.

DOSE: 1–8g dried herb equivalent three times daily.

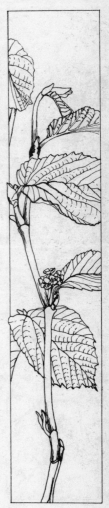

Harpogophytum procumbens

(Pedaliaceae)

DEVIL'S CLAW, TEUFELSKRALLE, DUIWELSKLOU

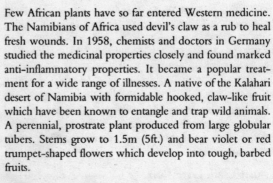

Few African plants have so far entered Western medicine. The Namibians of Africa used devil's claw as a rub to heal fresh wounds. In 1958, chemists and doctors in Germany studied the medicinal properties closely and found marked anti-inflammatory properties. It became a popular treatment for a wide range of illnesses. A native of the Kalahari desert of Namibia with formidable hooked, claw-like fruit which have been known to entangle and trap wild animals. A perennial, prostrate plant produced from large globular tubers. Stems grow to 1.5m (5ft.) and bear violet or red trumpet-shaped flowers which develop into tough, barbed fruits.

PARTS USED: Tuber.

ACTIVE INGREDIENTS/ACTIONS: Iridoid glycosides, including harpagoside, harpagide and procumbide; flavonoids, especially kaempferol and luteolin glycosides; phenolic acids. Anti-inflammatory, anti-rheumatic, analgesic, sedative.

MEDICINAL USE: Useful in rheumatism, arthritis, gout, myalgia, fibrositis and lumbago, for which it is a specific. **Warning:** Should not be used in pregnancy as it may stimulate uterine muscle.

PREPARATIONS: Decoction, tincture.

DOSE: 1–10g dried root equivalent three times daily.

Humulus lupulus
(Cannabinaceae)

HOPS

Hops were first used as a vegetable in ancient Greece. They are best known as a flavour in beer-making. It was first used for ale in the fourteenth century in Holland, reaching Britain only in the sixteenth century, where it was at first banned by Henry VI. The local taste was for ales flavoured with ground ivy, wormwood, yarrow, or marjoram and the use of hops was seen as a sacrilege. After accepting hops in ale, their medicinal uses were appreciated. John Evelyn, the diarist, wrote in 1670 that hops in ale 'preserves the drink indeed, but repays the pleasure in tormenting diseases and a shorter life'. A native of Britain but now found in most temperate lands. A perennial climber with heart-shaped, lobed leaves with finely toothed margins. Male and female flowers are on separate plants and appear in late summer. The male type are in loose bunches and the female, which is the part used in brewing, are yellowish-green cone-like catkins 3–4cm (1.5in.) long. The inner leaves of the catkins bear visible oil glands. The smell is strong and characteristic. Easily cultivated.

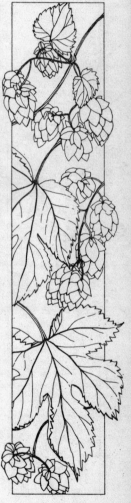

PARTS USED: Female flowers or strobiles.

ACTIVE INGREDIENTS/ACTIONS: Volatile oil, mainly humulene; flavonols, including glycosides of quercetin, kaempferol; resin; tannin; oestrogenic substances. Sedative, tranquillizer, hypnotic, antispasmodic, diuretic, bitter.

MEDICINAL USE: As a sedative in insomnia except where depression is involved; for relief of nervous stomach conditions including irritable bowel. **Warning:** Hops are an anaphrodisiac for men.

PREPARATIONS: Infusion, hop pillows, tablets, tincture.

DOSE: 1–4g dried strobile equivalent three times daily.

Hydrastis canadensis

(Ranunculaceae)

GOLDEN SEAL, HYDRASTIS, ORANGE ROOT

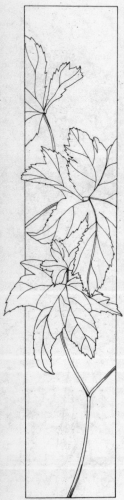

The alkaloids in golden seal are among the most useful in the herbalist's pharmacy. The Native Americans used it as a specific herb for vaginal inflammations and for external ulceration or wounds. It was also a useful yellow dye for cloth and face decoration. The white settlers took up the herb so enthusiastically that its collection from the wild almost caused its extinction. Now it is protected and commercial supplies come only from cultivation. Native to North America, in cool shady woods. A small perennial arising from a large rhizome and sending up a flowering stem to 30cm (12in.) bearing two five-lobed, serrated leaves. The flower appears in spring in the angle of a leaf. It is indistinct with no petals and develops into a raspberry-like fruit. Easily cultivated.

PARTS USED: Rhizome and roots.

ACTIVE INGREDIENTS/ACTIONS: Alkaloids including hydrastine, berberine, and canadine; volatile oil; resin. Astringent and vulnerary to mucous membranes throughout the body; digestive stimulant, cholagogue.

MEDICINAL USE: Useful for intestinal inflammations including gastritis, peptic ulcers, enteritis; a douche for vaginal infections including thrush and trichonomas; as a mouthwash for aphthous ulcers and gingivitis; for topical use on wounds and eruptions including boils and carbuncles. **Warning:** Avoid in pregnancy and high blood pressure.

PREPARATIONS: Decoction, tincture, tablets.

DOSE: 0.5–2g dried root equivalent three times daily.

Hyoscyamus niger

(Solanaceae)

HENBANE, HOG'S BEAN, CASSILATA

Although a close relative of the tomato and potato, henbane is a deadly poison when abused. It has been used as both a medicine and a poison for centuries. Shakespeare knew of henbane. A little of 'the leprous distillment' of henbane was poured into the ear of Hamlet's father while he slept and it killed him. It has been used for various medicinal uses including as a painkiller and a head lice poison. The plant was used as a dried herb, juice, and the leaves were smoked. Native to Europe but naturalized in both Americas and Australasia. An annual or biennial growing to 1.5m (5ft.) with an erect stem sprouting jointed hairs. Leaves are long, ovate, hairy and sticky. Brown or yellow flowers with purple veins appear in summer in the leaf axils. Easily cultivated.

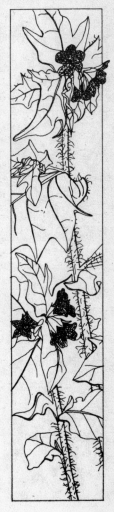

PARTS USED: Leaves, especially during flowering.

ACTIVE INGREDIENTS/ACTIONS: Tropane alkaloids, especially hyoscyamine, hyoscine, scopalamine. Antispasmodic, sedative, anticholinergic.

MEDICINAL USE: Valuable for bronchial spasm or asthma; an antispasmodic for the intestinal tract and urinary tubules in colic. **Warning:** Not be used except by health professionals.

PREPARATIONS: Herbal cigarettes, tincture.

DOSE: Dose must not exceed 100mg leaf equivalent three times daily.

Hypericum perforatum

(Hyperaceae)

ST JOHN'S WORT

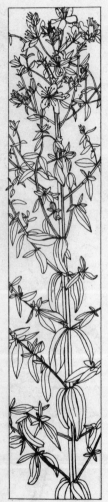

Not to be confused with St James' wort (*Senecio jacobaea*) or St John's herb (*Eupatorium canabium*). The Greek name *Hypericum* comes from the herb's legendary magical properties, which included chasing away the devil. The common name is from either the property of the yellow petals turning to red when crushed or the time of flowering, which coincides with the date St John was beheaded, 24 June. A native of Europe and Asia but widely naturalized. A perennial with thin, erect woody stems growing to 60cm (23.5in.) and having two raised opposite ridges or wings. Leaves are hairless, oblong and have distinct, transparent oil glands looking like perforations when held to the light. Apical clusters of five-petalled, yellow flowers appear in early summer. Cultivation easy.

PARTS USED: Herb, including flowers.

ACTIVE INGREDIENTS/ACTIONS: Essential oil with caryophyllene, pinene, limonene and myrcene; hypericins; flavonoids; resin. Sedative, astringent, anxiolytic, antidepressant, anti-inflammatory, topically antiseptic.

MEDICINAL USE: An established antidepressant; useful in excitability and mild anxiety; externally for wounds, burns and infections.

PREPARATIONS: Infusion, tincture, infused red oil made from steeped flowers.

DOSE: 2–10g dried herb equivalent three times daily.

Hyssopus officinalis
(Labitae)

HYSSOP

An ancient European herb that has had associations with religious ceremonies and traditional medicines. It was one of the strewing herbs that were scattered on the floors of houses to repel insects. Medicinally used to kill head lice and internal worms as well as for its more traditional role in easing colds and coughs. Native to Europe and western Asia. Widely naturalized and grown in gardens, especially on alkaline soils in sunny positions. A highly aromatic perennial to 60cms (24in.) high with thin pointed leaves covered in fine hairs. Small blue flowers appear in whorls around leaf axils in late summer. Easily cultivated.

PARTS USED: Herb.

ACTIVE INGREDIENTS/ACTIONS: Volatile oil with pinocamphone, camphor, thujone, pinene, linalool; terpenoids including marrubiin, oleanolic, ursolic acids; flavonoids; tannin. Diaphoretic, expectorant, carminative, sedative.

MEDICINAL USE: An excellent calming expectorant; used in bronchitis, chronic nasal catarrh, coughs and colds.

PREPARATIONS: Infusion, tincture.

DOSE: 2-10g dried herb equivalent three times daily.

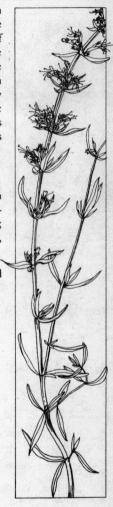

Inula helenium

(Compositae)

ELECAMPANE, SCABWORT, HORSEHEAL, AUNEÉ, ALANTWURZEL.

Elecampane was used by the ancient Greeks and Romans as a digestive tonic after their reputedly indulgent feasting. It is believed that the generic name is after Helen of Troy. It used to be a popular plant in European gardens as a medicine and a confection, after being candied. Native to Europe and found in damp pastures and roadsides. A perennial to 2m (6.5ft.) with a deep taproot and hairy erect stems with large elliptical leaves having hairy undersides. Flower-heads appear in late summer and have many slender bright yellow ray florets. Easily cultivated.

PARTS USED: Root.

ACTIVE INGREDIENTS/ACTIONS: Volatile oil with sesquiterpene lactones including helanin, and derivatives like azulene; inulin. Stimulating expectorant, diaphoretic, digestive, bacteriostatic.

MEDICINAL USE: Used in bronchial and other respiratory conditions with resistant catarrh and a persistent cough; cough in tuberculosis; irritating cough in children.

PREPARATIONS: Infusion, tincture.

DOSE: 2–10g dried root equivalent three times daily.

Lactuca virosa

(Compositae)

WILD LETTUCE, LETTUCE OPIUM, LAITUE VIREUSE

The wild parent of domesticated salad lettuce. The common name 'poor man's opium' hints at the opiate-like ingredients and not the effects of taking the herb. The white latex, known as lactucarium, was used in the nineteenth century as an adulterant for opium. A traditional ingredient in cough mixtures where it acts as a sedative and cough suppressant. Native to Europe. This biennial plant has a slightly raised rosette of leaves, which are ovate, covered in stout hairs and up to 30cms (12in.) long. In the second year, an erect flowering stem rises up to 1.8m (6ft.), bearing numerous short-stalked, yellow, daisy-like flowers. The plant has a strong odour and all parts exude a white latex when cut. Easily cultivated.

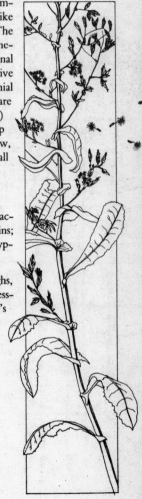

PARTS USED: Leaves.

ACTIVE INGREDIENTS/ACTIONS: The sesquiterpene lactone, lactucin; flavonoids including quercetin; coumarins; an alkaloid thought to be hyoscyamine. Sedative, hypnotic, mild anodyne.

MEDICINAL USE: Used in bronchitis, irritable coughs, insomnia especially in children with anxiety and restlessness. **Warning:** To be used only under a herbalist's supervision as overdose can produce stupor, even coma and death.

PREPARATIONS: Infusion, tincture.

DOSE: 0.5–5g dried herb equivalent three times daily.

Lavandula angustifolia

(Labitae)

LAVENDER

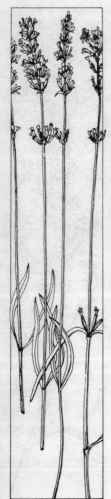

One of the best known and loved herbs since Roman times. It has been used as a perfume, insect repellent, flavourer of foods and medicine. Entered in the British pharmacopoeia for over 250 years and has been recorded in medicinal use for longer. Its earliest citation said it was useful for 'the Falling sickness, and all cold Dis-tempers of the Head, Womb, Stomach and Nerves; against the Apoplexy, Palsy, Convulsions, Megrim, Vertigo, Loss of Memory, Dimness of Sight, Melancholy, Swooning Fits and Barrenness in Women'. Native to southern and western Europe around the Mediterranean. A woody perennial shrub with opposite and very narrow leaves which are grey-green and covered in fine hair. Blue-violet and highly perfumed flowers appear on spikes in mid to late summer. Easily cultivated.

PARTS USED: Flowers, distilled oil.

ACTIVE INGREDIENTS/ACTIONS: Volatile oil with linalyl acetate, linalool, borneol, camphor, limonene; coumarins; flavonoids. Carminative, spasmolytic, nervous tonic.

MEDICINAL USE: A general nervous system relaxant, especially in baths, to relieve irritability, insomnia, exhaustion and depression. A digestive tonic and carminative in flatulence; used topically to relieve tension headaches and arthritic or spastic muscular pains.

PREPARATIONS: Volatile oil, tincture.

DOSE: 1–8g dried flowers equivalent three times daily.

Leonorus cardica

(Labitae)

MOTHERWORT, LION'S EAR

The herb most often given the properties of 'gladdening and strengthening the heart'. The ancient Greeks used it to calm the nervousness of new mothers and to relax the body in menopause. It also reduces the palpitations and irregular heartbeats sometimes created by nervous tension and anxiety. A European native, which has been widely naturalized, it prefers alkaline, dry soils. Unlike other members of the *Labitae*, it has deeply lobed leaves and a prickly base to the flowers. It is perennial with typical square stems and hairs on leaves and stem. Leaves are closely spaced up the erect stem with pink–blue flowers in whorls in the leaf axils during midsummer. Easily cultivated.

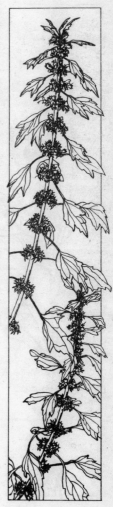

PARTS USED: Herb.

ACTIVE INGREDIENTS/ACTIONS: Iridoids including leonuride; diterpenes; flavonoids including rutin, quercetin, hyperoside, apigenin. Mild uterine stimulant, relaxant, antispasmodic, cardiac tonic, mildly hypotensive.

MEDICINAL USE: Used for general nervous tension, and for palpitations and tachycardia. Helpful in painful periods with nervous tension or anxiety and in flushing and night sweats in menopause.

PREPARATIONS: Infusion, tincture, tablets.

DOSE: 2–8g dried herb equivalent three times daily.

Lobelia inflata

(Lobeliaceae)

LOBELIA, PUKEWEED, INDIAN TOBACCO

The common name suggests the powerful emetic action of this herb that was one of the most important medicines used by the North American Physiomedical School of Herbalists in the nineteenth century. Native Americans smoked lobelia to cure their asthma and related respiratory problems. The herb was introduced to Europe in 1929. A native of North America and widely introduced from there. It is annual or biennial with a hairy, erect stem to 60cm (2ft.) with alternate oval to oblong leaves which are without petioles and have a finely toothed margin. Flowers are blue in loose terminal racemes in the summer. A small round capsule containing two seeds is produced. Easily cultivated.

PARTS USED: Herb.

ACTIVE INGREDIENTS/ACTIONS: Alkaloids, including lobeline, isolobeline, lobelanidine; chelidonic acid; volatile oil, lobelianin; resin; gum. Respiratory stimulant, antiasthmatic, antispasmodic, emetic (in large doses).

MEDICINAL USE: For asthma and chronic bronchitis with tightness; locally in rheumatic and muscular inflammation; the emetic effect is used to help break nicotine addiction. **Warning:** Should be used only under the supervision of a qualified practitioner.

PREPARATIONS: Herbal cigarettes, infusion, tincture.

DOSE: 0.02–0.08g dried herb equivalent three times daily. Maximum permitted dose in UK is 100mg dried herb equivalent three times daily.

Marrubrium vulgare

(Labitae)

WHITE HOREHOUND, HOARHOUND

For centuries, traditional cough remedies have included this herb. It is one of the most reliable cough remedies known and is in cough prescriptions used by the Egyptian pharaohs. *Marrubrium* has been used as an antidote to various poisons from arrows to the bitings of mad dogs. Its social importance is evident in its inclusion among the list of bitter herbs that should be eaten at the Feast of Passover. A native of Europe where it grows on roadsides and waste places. A perennial with hairy square stems and ovate leaves, which are much wrinkled and feel leathery. Small white flowers appear in tight whorls in leaf axils during summer and produce tightly packed seeds in an urn-shaped receptacle. Easily cultivated.

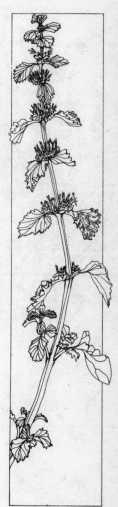

PARTS USED: Herb, collected during flowering.

ACTIVE INGREDIENTS/ACTIONS: Sesquiterpene bitters, marrubiin; volatile oil with pinene, sabine, camphene, cymol; alkaloids; tannins. Stimulating expectorant, bitter tonic, antiseptic, circulatory stimulant.

MEDICINAL USE: Used in chronic catarrhal colds and bronchitis; useful in pertussis; and as a cholagogue.

PREPARATIONS: Infusion, tincture, pharmaceutical preparations.

DOSE: 2–8g dried herb equivalent three times daily.

Matricaria recutita

(Compositae) also *M. chamomilla*

GERMAN CHAMOMILE, WILD CHAMOMILE

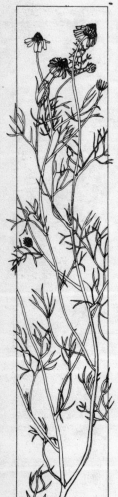

Not a true botanical chamomile, which it closely resembles. One of the most ancient of plant medicines. It is drunk all around the world as a calming digestive tea or tisane. Known as the plant's physician and used as a companion plant to cure and prevent diseases. Its many medicinal uses have been confirmed by scientific experiments and clinical trials. Native to Europe and North Africa. A low-growing, tufted perennial with finely divided leaves and yellow-centred daisy-like flowers with white rays. It is distinguished from the true chamomiles by the hollow, conical centre to the flower and the absence of the small chaffy scales between adjacent yellow florets on the cone. Cultivated with care.

PARTS USED: Flowers.

ACTIVE INGREDIENTS/ACTIONS: Volatile oil, azulene, containing chamazulene, matricine and bisabolol; flavonoids, apigenin, luteolin, quercetin; coumarins. Antispasmodic, sedative, antifungal, antibacterial, analgesic, vulnerary, carminative, bitter.

MEDICINAL USE: A mild, relaxing sedative for adults and children; used for gastritis and irritated stomach or intestines; gently calming for nervous stomach and in irritable bowel; helps relieve pain in periods, migraine, rheumatism and gout; an excellent topical remedy to ease allergic dermatitis including eczema when tea bags can be applied; helps heal burns and weeping wounds. Some people dislike the aroma and can feel nauseous.

PREPARATIONS: Infusion, tincture, essential oil, creams.

DOSE: 2–8g dried flower equivalent three times daily.

Melaleuca leucadendron

(Myrtaceae)

CAJAPUT, SWAMP TEA-TREE, PAPERBARK TEA-TREE

One of the several families of Australian trees rich in aromatic oils, especially cineol, that are world-famous in cold and headache medicines. The eucalyptus or gum trees are from the same family. Used by the Australian Aborigines for 30,000 years as a local painkiller by rubbing leaves between the hands and then running them over the affected parts. Crushed leaves and sometimes hot infusions were sniffed to relieve headaches. A related tree *M. alternifolia* is the source of the strongly antiseptic tea-tree oil. Native to Australia and South East Asia, growing in swampy light soils near the coasts. An evergreen tree to 35m(115ft.) with slender, hairy leaves, and papery, cream bark. Flowers appear in summer as a spike around stem ends. Difficult to cultivate.

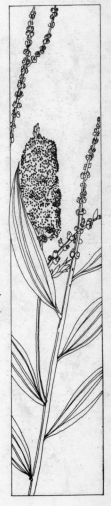

PARTS USED: Leaves.

ACTIVE INGREDIENTS/ACTIONS: Volatile oil containing cineole, alpha terpineol. Stimulant, antispasmodic, expectorant, anodyne.

MEDICINAL USE: Used in coughs and colds to relieve blocked sinuses, and catarrhal chests and asthma; in relief of toothache and headache; to calm colic and stomach cramps; useful as a rubifacient in rheumatism, sprains and muscle strains.

PREPARATIONS: Essential oil, pharmaceutical preparations.

DOSE: 0.05-0.02ml essential oil.

Melilotus officinalis

(Leguminosae)

MELILOT, RIBED MELILOT, KING'S CLOVER

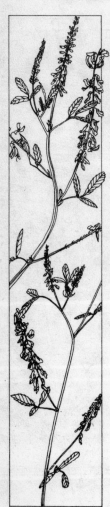

Once a common pasture plant in Britain and Europe, the herb is now found as a naturalized member of the local flora. The name comes from honey bees' preference for the flowers. Like woodruff, melilot has the aroma of freshly mown hay due to one ingredient, coumarin. A native of southern Europe and western Asia it is now widely naturalized. A perennial herb growing to 0.5m (1½ft.) high. Leaves are trifoliate, with oval leaflets. Racemes of perfumed, yellow flowers appear in summer and produce thin, wrinkled, black seed pods. Easily cultivated.

PARTS USED: Herb, during flowering.

ACTIVE INGREDIENTS/ACTIONS: Coumarins, dicoumarol, flavonoids, tannin. Anticoagulant, anti-inflammatory, carminative.

MEDICINAL USE: Used mainly in vascular problems with inflammation and increased risk of thrombosis.

PREPARATIONS: Infusion, tincture.

DOSE: 2-8g dried herb equivalent three times daily.

Melissa officinalis

(Labitae)

LEMON BALM, BALM, CURE ALL, SWEET BALM

The ancients used balm as a general remedy for an exhausted or befuddled nervous system. It was said it could 'renew youth, strengthen the brain, relieve languishing nature and prevent baldness'. John Evelyn said it would strengthen the brain and dispel melancholy, two symptoms reminiscent of anxiety and mild depression. Native to southern Europe but widely dispersed and a common garden herb world-wide. A perennial with a dense crown putting up slightly hairy stems to 1m (3ft.) bearing opposite, ovate, yellowish-green leaves with a rough surface and crenate margins. Crushed leaves have a strong lemon scent. Whitish flowers appear in late summer at stem apices and are attractive to bees. Easily cultivated.

PARTS USED: Fresh leaves.

ACTIVE INGREDIENTS/ACTIONS: Volatile oil with citral, linalool, citronellal, nerol, geraniol; flavonoids; polyphenols including caffeic and rosmarinic acids. Carminative, sedative, antispasmodic, diaphoretic, antiviral.

MEDICINAL USE: Used in anxiety states or to relieve nervous tension and associated insomnia; useful as a carminative; hot water infusions are used topically for herpes infections.

PREPARATIONS: Infusion (fresh herb), tincture.

DOSE: 15–30g fresh herb three times daily.

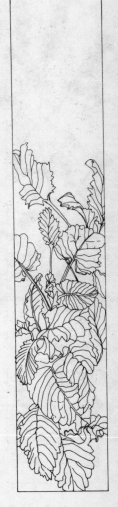

Mentha piperita

(Labitae)

PEPPERMINT

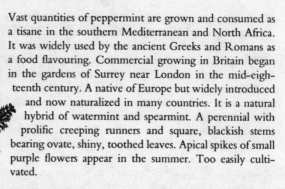

Vast quantities of peppermint are grown and consumed as a tisane in the southern Mediterranean and North Africa. It was widely used by the ancient Greeks and Romans as a food flavouring. Commercial growing in Britain began in the gardens of Surrey near London in the mid-eighteenth century. A native of Europe but widely introduced and now naturalized in many countries. It is a natural hybrid of watermint and spearmint. A perennial with prolific creeping runners and square, blackish stems bearing ovate, shiny, toothed leaves. Apical spikes of small purple flowers appear in the summer. Too easily cultivated.

PARTS USED: Herb.

ACTIVE INGREDIENTS/ACTIONS: Volatile oil with menthol, menthone, menthyl acetate, pinene, limonene, cineole; flavonoids, including rutin; azulene; rosmarinic acid. Spasmolytic, carminative, anti-emetic, diaphoretic, antiseptic.

MEDICINAL USE: A calming digestive in dyspepsia; relieves nausea from overeating or in early pregnancy; also useful in irritable bowel syndrome, colic and flatulence.

PREPARATIONS: Infusion, oil, tincture.

DOSE: 2–8g dried herb equivalent three times daily.

Menyanthes trifoliata

(Menyanthaceae)

BOGBEAN, BUCKBEAN, MARSH TREFOIL

Not a member of the bean family but a relative of gentian. It used to be used against scurvy, gout and rheumatism but is now used more as a substitute for the bitter, *Gentiana*. A native of Europe where it is found in shallow boggy ponds. A perennial with a creeping rootstock and trifoliate leaves, sheathed at the base. Flowers appear in midsummer as shaggy white-centred flowers with pinkish outers. Easily cultivated in ponds.

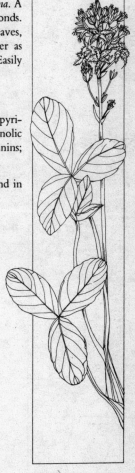

PARTS USED: Leaves.

ACTIVE INGREDIENTS/ACTIONS: Iridoid glycosides; pyridine alkaloids, including gentianine; coumarins; phenolic acids as caffeic and vanillic acids; vitamin C; tannins; flavonoids. Bitter, choleretic, diuretic.

MEDICINAL USE: Used in rheumatism, indigestion and in anorexia.

PREPARATIONS: Infusion, tincture.

DOSE: 1–4g dried herb equivalent three times daily.

Mitchella repens

(Rubiaceae)

SQUAW VINE, CHECKERBERRY, PARTRIDGE BERRY, WINTER
CLOVER, DEER BERRY.

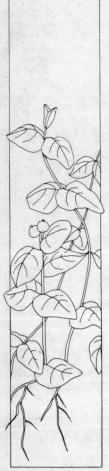

A Native American Indian remedy taken by pregnant
squaws in the final weeks to make the birth easier. A
native of eastern North America, where it grows in
woods. A small perennial herb with opposite, ovate leaves
with smooth margins and a bitter taste. Small white flowers appear at branch ends in summer and give way to red
berries. Cultivatable.

PARTS USED: Herb.

ACTIVE INGREDIENTS/ACTIONS: Saponins; mucilage;
tannins. Parturient, astringent, uterine relaxant, nervous
tonic.

MEDICINAL USE: To ease labour; helpful in dysmenorrhoea; useful in nervous exhaustion and irritability.

PREPARATIONS: Infusion, tincture.

DOSE: 8g dried herb equivalent three times daily.

Oenothera biennis

(Onagraceae)

EVENING PRIMROSE, TREE PRIMROSE, EVENING STAR

The seed oil is a rich, but not uniquely so, source of the fatty acid called gamma-linolenic acid. This is an essential fatty acid for health and in higher amounts has proved an effective treatment for atopic eczema, premenstrual syndrome, and thrombus formation or blood clotting. A native of North America but introduced into Europe in the early seventeenth century. It is now naturalized in many areas and a common garden plant. A biennial with a thick, deep, yellow taproot sprouting a basal rosette of long, oval leaves in the first year. The second year finds a vertical hairy stem to 1.5m (5ft.) with alternate lanceolate, soft leaves with short hairs. Flowers appear from midsummer as spikes in branches and are aromatic, yellow blooms to 5cm (2in.) in diameter. Flowers open in the evening. Easily cultivated.

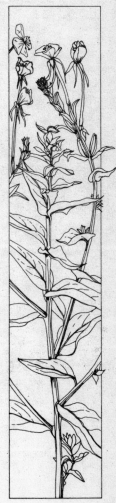

PARTS USED: Seed oil.

ACTIVE INGREDIENTS/ACTIONS: Fixed oil containing cis-linolenic acid and cis-γ-linolenic (GLA); Prostaglandin intermediary.

MEDICINAL USE: Oil is used internally and externally in atopic eczema, in premenstrual syndrome, excessive clotting tendency in heart and in vascular disease. Leaves have been used as a poultice.

PREPARATIONS: Oil, capsules.

DOSE: 200–600mg oil daily.

Origanum marjorana

(Labitae)

SWEET MARJORAM, ANNUAL OR KNOTTED MARJORAM

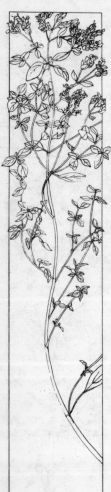

A treasured culinary herb that is closely related to oregano (*O. vulgare*) and wild marjorams. As with most culinary herbs, it was originally used as a medicine. In Greece, a popular 'stomach tea' called *Ditany* or *Dictamus*, which is a relative of marjoram, is as popular as mint or lime flower teas in northern Europe and North America. A native of North Africa and Central Asia but now widely distributed. A perennial in its natural habitat but grown as an annual in cooler climes. It has square, much branched and hairy stems. Leaves are elliptical, and opposite with entire margins. Flowers appear in mid to late summer as small condensed spikes of pinkish to purple small flowers. Easily cultivated.

PARTS USED: Herb harvested during flowering.

ACTIVE INGREDIENTS/ACTIONS: Volatile oil with sabinine, linalool, terpineol, eugenol; flavonoids including luteolin, apigenin derivatives; Phenolic acids, rosmarinic, caffeic; vitamin A. Stimulant, carminative, antispasmodic, emmenagogue.

MEDICINAL USE: A gentle carminative, usually taken in food.

PREPARATIONS: Dried herb.

DOSE: 10g dried herb equivalent three times daily.

Panax ginseng
(Araliaceae)

CHINESE GINSENG, ORIENTAL GINSENG, GINSENG

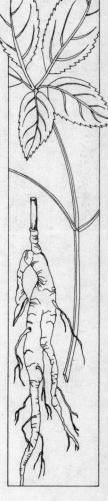

A common Chinese herb found in many health food shop products. The name 'ginseng' comes from the Chinese, 'renshen', meaning 'man root', because the thick, branched taproot can look like a man's legs. The Latin name means 'cure all'. The properties, which include stimulating the central nervous system, reducing fatigue, and increasing resistance to disease are exaggerated and many people take excessive amounts of the drug. The best quality ginseng is from Manchuria. American ginseng, *P. quinqufolium*, has fewer medical uses than the Oriental species. (See also *Elutherococcus senticosus*.) The high price of the best quality product has encouraged the sale of poor quality and diluted ginseng to the unwary. A perennial with a divided taproot sending up a single stem to 50cm (20in.) with up to 5 palmate leaves, each with thin, serrate, pointed leaflets. Flowers are small, greenish umbels that appear in late summer. Easily cultivated.

PARTS USED: Root.

ACTIVE INGREDIENTS/ACTIONS: Triterpene saponins called ginsenosides; glycosides, sterols, volatile oil. Both stimulant and relaxant on central nervous system, adrenogenic, improve muscle stamina, cardiotonic, hypoglycaemic, adaptogenic.

MEDICINAL USE: Useful in debility after illness or in old age; can increase concentration and stamina for short periods; improve body's response to stress. Should not be used for more than three weeks by the fit and active and should not be taken in acute inflammatory disease or in depression and anxiety states.

PREPARATIONS: Powdered root, tablets, tincture.

DOSE: 0.5-2g dried root equivalent three times daily.

Papaver somniferum

(Papaveraceae)

WHITE POPPY, OPIUM POPPY, MAWSEED

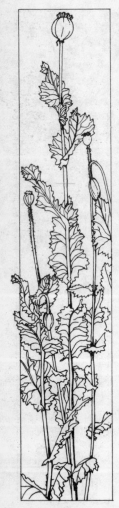

The earliest recorded use of the opium poppy was as a medicine. It was used by the Arabian physicians, who introduced opium to Europe, as well as by Indian, Greek and Roman physicians. Both morphine and codeine, two valuable pharmaceutical painkillers, derive from the opium poppy. The crude drug is 'tapped' by scratching the surface of the seed capsules when the petals have fallen and harvesting the exuding latex when it has dried. Native to the Middle East and western Asia but introduced elsewhere. An annual with silvery grey-green dentate leaves on unbranched stems. Flowers are from white to lilac, appear in midsummer, and are borne on large, globular capsules which ripen with a flattened top. All parts of the plant exude a white latex when scratched. Easily cultivated.

PARTS USED: Latex, leaves.

ACTIVE INGREDIENTS/ACTIONS: Alkaloids, especially morphine, codeine, papaverine, narcotine, sanguinarine. Narcotic, hypnotic, analgesic, antispasmodic, antidiarrhoeal, antitussive.

MEDICINAL USE: Common in pharmaceutical drugs to relieve diarrhoea and prevent coughs. It is used as a pre-operative relaxant while the extracted morphine is used in severe pain.

PREPARATIONS: Tincture, opium extract, pharmaceutical drugs.

DOSE: It is illegal to use the extracted latex.

Passiflora incarnata

(Passifloraceae)

PASSION FLOWER, MAYPOP, GRANADILLA

The common name is not a promise of aphrodisiac properties but a reference to the shape of the flower. The
beautiful and complex flower has an intricately sculptured
corona in the centre, which resembles Christ's crown of
thorns. A native of North America it is grown throughout
the world. It thrives on rich soils in sunny positions. A
perennial vine with a woody and slightly hairy stem.
Leaves are three-lobed, pointed, with serrate margins.
The related *P. caerulea* is illustrated. Flowers are cream
with purple centres and give way to orange, oval fruits
containing the seeds embedded in a scented and edible
pulp. Easily cultivated.

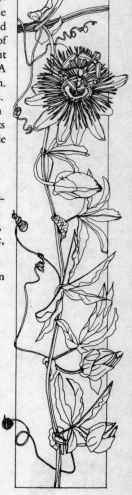

PARTS USED: Leaves.

ACTIVE INGREDIENTS/ACTIONS: Alkaloids including harman, harmine, harmaline, harmol, passiflorine; flavonoids
including apigenin, kaempferol, luteolin, quercetin, rutin,
saponarin; sterols. Sedative, hypnotic, antispasmodic,
hypotensive, anodyne.

MEDICINAL USE: A safe, gentle and non-addictive help in
restlessness, insomnia and nervous irritability.

PREPARATIONS: Infusion, tablets, tincture.

DOSE: 1–4g dried herb equivalent three times daily.

Phytolacca decandra
(Phytolaccaeae) also *P. americanana*

POKE ROOT, PIGEON BERRY, RED PLANT, POCAN, CANCER ROOT, AMERICAN NIGHTSHADE

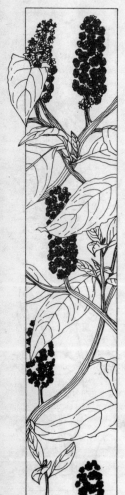

A Native American drug used originally to treat venereal disease. It is one of the more useful alteratives in Western herbal medicine. Leaves and seedlings have been eaten as a vegetable. The berries were reputed to be a cure for skin cancers. It came to Europe in the nineteenth century. A perennial with a thick, deep-purple stem to 3m (10ft.) with alternate oblong to spear-shaped leaves having a strong smell. Flowers are white to pink on a tight, terminal raceme and are followed by round, soft, purple berries. A native of south and east United States on rich, light soils in open country. Easily cultivated.

PARTS USED: Root, berries.

ACTIVE INGREDIENTS/ACTIONS: Triterpenoid saponins or phytolaccosides; alkaloid, phytolaccine; lectins, known as mitogen. Alterative, anti-inflammatory, immune stimulant, lymphatic, antirheumatic, paraciticide, antifungal.

MEDICINAL USE: Widely indicated for glandular, toxic and metabolic disorders; in rheumatic disease; inflammatory disease of the respiratory system; to conditions where the lymphatic system needs stimulating; in skin disease. **Warning:** Large doses may be cathartic and emetic. Should be used only on the advice of a qualified practitioner.

PREPARATIONS: Tincture.

DOSE: 0.05–0.5g dried root equivalent three times daily.

Picrasma excelsia

(Simarubaceae) also *Quassia amara*

QUASSIA, BITTER WOOD, JAMAICA QUASSIA

In recognition of the Third World origins of many of our most useful medicines, this plant was named after the Guyanan slave, Quassi, who taught Europeans how to use the plant to treat tropical fevers. It is also an insecticide especially potent when used against flies and mites. Native to the West Indies, especially Jamaica, St Vincent and Antigua. It is a tall tree growing to 20m (65ft.) with pinnate leaves like an ash, with small greenish flowers appearing in late summer and producing bunches of small black fruits. Difficult to cultivate.

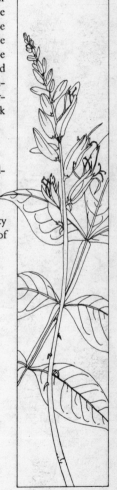

PARTS USED: Wood.

ACTIVE INGREDIENTS/ACTIONS: Bitter quassinoids including quassin, isoquassin or picrasmin; alkaloids; scopoletin; sitosterol. Tonic, bitter, anthelmintic, antimalarial.

MEDICINAL USE: A general bitter tonic used in debility with poor digestion and appetite; useful in infestations of amoebae, threadworms and nematodes.

PREPARATIONS: Decoctions of wood chips, tincture.

DOSE: 0.3–0.6g dried bark equivalent three times daily.

Piscidia erythrina

(Leguminosae)

JAMAICA DOGWOOD, FISH POISON BARK

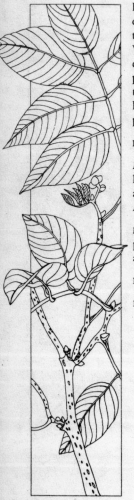

In the Caribbean and Central America, the leaves are crushed and the released juices washed into rivers or ponds to stun fish, which float to the surface for easy collection. Warm-blooded animals are unaffected. The plant also contains rotenone, which is used as an insecticide. This plant illustrates how animal species can react differently to the same drugs. Native to Central America. A small legiminous tree or shrub with longitudinal wings on its pods. Difficult to cultivate.

PARTS USED: Bark.

ACTIVE INGREDIENTS/ACTIONS: Isoflavones including lisetin, jamacin; rotenoids including rotenone, milletone and isomilletone; piscidic acid; sitosterol; tannins. Analgesic, sedative, antispasmodic.

MEDICINAL USE: Used for insomnia, neuralgia, headache, period pains. **Warning:** Should be taken only on the advice of a qualified practitioner.

PREPARATIONS: Tincture.

DOSE: 0.5–4g dried herb equivalent three times daily.

Plantago major

(Plantaginaceae) also *P. lanceolata, P. ovata*

GREATER PLANTAIN, RIBWORT, RAT'S TAIL PLANTAIN, ISBOGOOL, PSYLLIUM

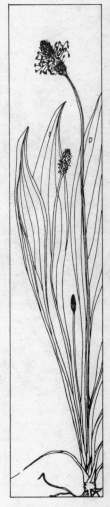

An ancient traditional remedy for wounds, easing irritable coughs and stopping diarrhoeas. It was one of the Saxons' nine sacred herbs. The seed husks of a related species *P. ovata* are effective bulking agents for both diarrhoea and constipation. These husks appear in pharmaceutical preparations like Fybogel. Plantain was the subject of superstitions that Gerard dismissed as 'but ridiculous toyes'. Native to Europe on rich grassland, but has spread around the world as a successful weed. A perennial with a basal rosette of slightly hairy leaves which vary from lanceolate to ovate and a familiar spike of small greenish flowers with tiny purple anthers which appear from midsummer. Easy to cultivate.

PARTS USED: Leaves, seeds.

ACTIVE INGREDIENTS/ACTIONS: *P. major:* Iridoids including acubin; flavonoids including apigenin, luteolin, scutellarin, baicalein; organic acids, including fumaric and benzoic; tannins. *P. ovata:* up to 30 per cent mucilage; triterpenes. Leaves are demulcent, astringent, expectorant, diuretic. *P. ovata* is bulk laxative.

MEDICINAL USE: Leaves are used in cystitis, in catarrhal conditions of the respiratory tract, locally for haemorrhoids. Psyllium husks are used as a bulk laxative and to reduce diarrhoea.

PREPARATIONS: Infusion, cream, tincture, solution of husks.

DOSE: 2–8g dried leaf equivalent three times daily; 5.25g dried husks 2–3 times daily.

Potentilla erecta

(Rosaceae) also *P. tormentilla*

TORMENTIL, BLOODROOT, EWE DAISY, SHEPHERD'S KNOT

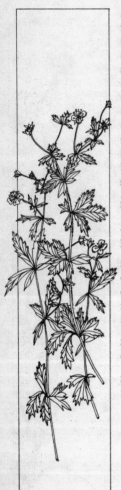

A humble and unassuming meadow herb with a stunning red pigment stored in its roots. It was a favourite traditional remedy, appearing in formulas for all manner of ailments from ague to cholera. The whole plant is highly astringent and was also used as a therapeutic tooth powder to ease bleeding and infected gums and as an excellent treatment for external sores, ulcers and even piles. Native to northern Europe and West Asia on acid, damp soils in the lowlands. A short perennial with a thick, red-centred rootstock, and prostrate, wandering stems bearing five-lobed leaves with serrate, lanceolate segments. Flowers are bright yellow, four-petalled, appearing throughout the summer. Easily cultivated.

PARTS USED: Root, herb.

ACTIVE INGREDIENTS/ACTIONS: Tannins; red pigment, phlobaphene. Astringent.

MEDICINAL USE: A safe and effective astringent throughout the gut for gastritis, colitis, and diarrhoea; a more tolerable mouthwash than myrrh in gingivitis and throat infections; an effective vaginal douche in leucorrhoea; an ingredient in leg ulcer and pile creams and lotions.

PREPARATIONS: Decoction of root, infusion, tincture, creams.

DOSE: 2-6 dried roots or herb equivalent three times daily internally.

Prunella vulgaris

(Labiatae)

SELF–HEAL, SICLEWORT, HEAL ALL, HEART OF THE EARTH, HOOK HEAL

A favourite wound healing remedy from the Middle Ages. Gerard said that, together with its relative bugle (*Ajuga reptans*) 'in all the world there are not two better wound herbs, as has often been proved'. Its merits were aptly exemplified by Culpeper who said, it was 'Self-Heal, whereby when you are hurt, you may heal yourself'. Native to Europe but spread with colonization and trade and is now naturalized all round the world. A perennial with a creeping rhizome and a habit dependent on fertility. In poor soil it is creeping, but in rich soil it rises to 60cm (24in.) with square stems and opposite pairs at right angles to the preceding pair. Leaves are oblong with dentate margins and a shiny, dark–green surface. Flowers are violet in tight spikes appearing from midsummer. Easily cultivated.

PARTS USED: Herb.

ACTIVE INGREDIENTS/ACTIONS: Triterpenes derived from ursolic, betulinic and oleanolic acid; tannins. Astringent, styptic, vulnerary.

MEDICINAL USE: Used as a styptic and salve on open wounds; useful internally for bleeding and healing ulcers and sore throats.

PREPARATIONS: Infusion, poultice, tincture.

DOSE: 2–8g dried herb equivalent three times daily.

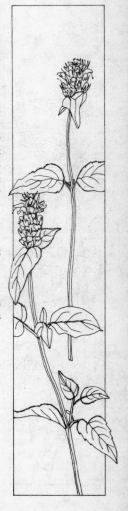

253

Prunus serotina

(Rosaceae)

WILD CHERRY, VIRGINIAN PRUNE BARK

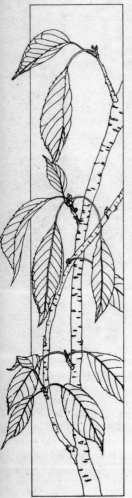

A close relative of the sloe and buckthorn, which have been used as rheumatic remedies. Wild cherry bark is one of the most useful cherry-based remedies in contemporary herbal medicine. It has been the base for cough and bronchitis medicines for the last 100 years. Native to North America. A large tree to 30m (98ft.) with alternate ovate leaves with dentate margins and clusters of white flowers in racemes during spring. The bark is smooth with rough lenticels, red-brown and shiny with a bitter astringent taste. It separates easily from the trunk. Easily cultivated.

PARTS USED: Bark or tree and roots.

ACTIVE INGREDIENTS/ACTIONS: Cyanogenic glycoside, prunasin; benzamdehyde; coumarins; tannins; resin. Antitussive, mild sedative, astringent.

MEDICINAL USE: Excellent for an irritable and unproductive cough; for bronchitis and unproductive nervous coughs.

PREPARATIONS: Bark, syrup, tincture.

DOSE: 2–8g dried bark equivalent three times daily.

Quercus robur

(Fagaceae)

OAK BARK, ENGLISH OAK, PEDUNCULATE OAK

The oak's medicinal credentials are as solid as its wood. It has ancient religious associations with the Greeks, Romans and Druids. The acorns have always been a valued pig food and have been gratefully eaten by human populations during famines. The mighty oak also provides dyes, used in tanning leather, and is one of the best astringent medicines. Galls, tannin rich growths produced by the tree in response to insect attack, are valued medicines because of their concentration of the astringent principles. A native to Europe, North Africa and West Asia but associated traditionally with England. It has been widely introduced. The tree can grow to enormous girth, spread and height (40m or 131ft.). Bark is smooth in youth but soon becomes rough and deeply furrowed. Leaves are familiar ovate with large lobes. Flowering is in summer, followed by acorns. Leaves are often deformed by galls caused by insects. Easily cultivated.

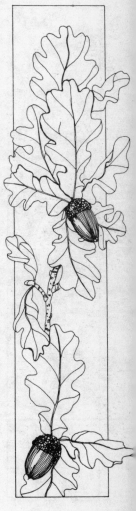

PARTS USED: Bark, galls.

ACTIVE INGREDIENTS/ACTIONS: Tannins including phlobatannin, ellagitannins and gallic acid. Astringent, styptic, antiseptic.

MEDICINAL USE: Used in acute diarrhoea; applied locally on burns and bleeding or weeping wounds; excellent for haemorrhoids; used as a mouthwash in gingivitis, aphthous ulcers; a vaginal douche.

PREPARATIONS: Decoction, tincture.

DOSE: 1–8g dried bark or gall equivalent three times daily.

Rosmarinus officinalis

(Labitae)

ROSEMARY, COMPASS PLANT

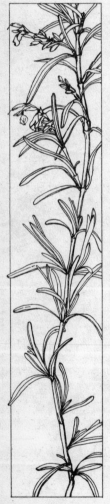

An ancient garden plant with a great legacy of mythical powers and reputed influences on life. It was used in weddings as a symbol of love and loyalty, often being incorporated in bridal wreaths. Rosemary is earnestly believed to grow strongly in the kitchen gardens of households where the woman rules supreme. It is a treasured plant for bee-keepers, making a particularly scented honey, and has been used to flavour both wine and ale. A widely appreciated culinary herb. A native of the northern shores of the Mediterranean but grown around the world. A shrub with distinct leathery, needle-like leaves with a bluey-green hue. Flowers appear as pink to blue racemes in leaf axils from spring to midsummer. Easily cultivated.

PARTS USED: Leaves.

ACTIVE INGREDIENTS/ACTIONS: Volatile oil with borneol, linalool, pinene, camphene, cineole, camphor; flavonoids, apigenin, diosmetin and diosmin; rosmarinic acid; tannins; resin. Circulatory stimulant, vasodilator, anti-inflammatory, astringent, nervine, antiseptic.

MEDICINAL USE: A stimulating nervine in exhaustion, depression, and debility; stimulant to peripheral circulation in migraines and skin disease; a rubifacient in liniments and lotions; useful where poor liver function is combined with poor circulation; useful as a hair rinse in dandruff and early hair loss.

PREPARATIONS: Infusion, juice, essential oil, tincture.

DOSE: 1–5g dried herb equivalent three times daily.

Rubus idaeus

(Rosaceae)

RASPBERRY

A wild food crop harvested during summer for centuries. It was one of the earliest of domesticated soft fruits and there are now hundreds of varieties, but little significant difference from the wild parents. Native to Europe and cultivated in many parts of the world. A thorny perennial behaving like a biennial. Suckers appearing one summer, flower and fruit the next. Stems bear dense prickle cover and leaves which are leathery on top and grey underneath with 3 to 5 leaflets. Flowers are small, appear in midsummer, and are followed by red cone-shaped fruit. Easily cultivated.

PARTS USED: Leaves.

ACTIVE INGREDIENTS/ACTIONS: Flavonoids including kaempferol, quercetin; polypeptides; tannins. Astringent, relaxing and toning to the pregnant uterus.

MEDICINAL USE: Used in last trimester of pregnancy to relax uterine muscles and facilitate birth; a gentle mouth gargle in minor throat and mucous membrane infections; an eyewash in conjunctivitis.

PREPARATIONS: Infusion, tincture.

DOSE: 2–8g dried herb equivalent three times daily.

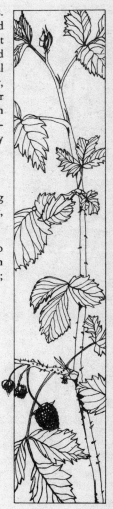

Rumex crispus

(Polygonaceae)

YELLOW DOCK, CURLED DOCK

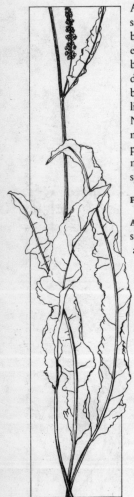

A close relative of sorrel, a tangy vegetable for soups and salads. The docks can also be eaten when young but are barely appealing. Docks have long been used for their effect on the liver and the bowel, for which they used to be the choice for purging. The ancient Romans also used docks for skin complaints. Gerard said it 'purifieth the blood and makes young wenches look fair and cherry-like', the former use referring to its value as a liver herb. Native to Europe but widespread and a common weed in many countries. A strong taproot sends up leaves with long petioles and ribbon-like leaves with an undulating or wavy margin. Flowers are small in whorls borne on a branched spike rising to 1m (3ft.) in midsummer. Easily cultivated.

PARTS USED: Root.

ACTIVE INGREDIENTS/ACTIONS: Anthraquinone glycosides; rumicin; oxalates; tannin. Aperient, laxative, alterative, cholagogue, bitter tonic.

MEDICINAL USE: A gentle laxative (aperient) especially in chronic atonic constipation; used in inflammatory skin disease where sluggish liver or bowel function is involved, especially eczemas, and psoriasis.

PREPARATIONS: Tincture, decoction.

DOSE: 1–8g dried root equivalent three times daily.

Salix alba

(Salicaceae)

WHITE WILLOW

An ancient traditional remedy for 'arthritis' and other bodily aches and pains. The active ingredients are anti-inflammatory. Salix is one of the sources of salicin, which led to the production of salicylic acid, commonly known as aspirin, still the most widely used pharmaceutical pain reliever. A native of Europe. This graceful tree grows to 25m (82ft.) with grey bark and long, slightly curved lanceolate, green leaves with a slightly downy surface. Flowers appear in early summer. Easily cultivated.

PARTS USED: Bark.

ACTIVE INGREDIENTS/ACTIONS: Phenolic glycosides including salicin, picein, triandrin with esters of salicylic acid; tannins; coumarins; flavonoids. Analgesic, anti-inflammatory, febrifuge, tonic.

MEDICINAL USE: Used in rheumatic pain in joints and muscles, gout, and in fever management; useful in enteritis and dysentery.

PREPARATIONS: Infusion, tincture.

DOSE: 2–8g dried bark equivalent three times daily.

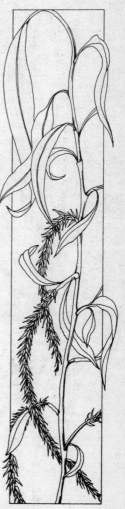

Salvia officinalis

(Labiatae)

RED SAGE, GARDEN SAGE, SPANISH SAGE

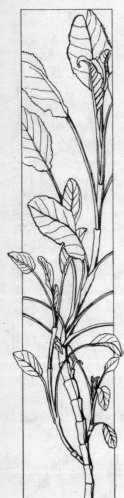

Sage has been a popular food and medicine throughout history. It has been used to flavour beer and cheese and remains a popular garden and kitchen herb. A popular tea or tisane. Its generic name comes from the Latin, *salvere*, to be saved, and it was said that having sage in the home garden meant no illness could prevail. Native to south-western Europe and the northern Mediterranean coast and hinterland, where it is grown prolifically. Many varieties exist and the plant changes its habit with the environment. It is a perennial shrub to 70cm (27in.) with rugose, glandular leaves which can be reddish or green and ovate. Violet flowers appear on terminal spikes in late summer to autumn. Easily cultivated.

PARTS USED: Leaves.

ACTIVE INGREDIENTS/ACTIONS: Volatile oil with thujone, cineole, borneol, camphor; diterpene bitters; flavonoids including salvigenin, genkwanin, luteolin; phenolic acids including rosmarinic and caffeic acids; oestrogenic substances; tannins. Astringent, anhydrotic, antiseptic, vulnerary, reduces salivation and lactation, uterine stimulant, cholagogue.

MEDICINAL USE: A general mouthwash for gingivitis, aphthous ulcers, and throat infections; a circulation stimulant; a bitter for digestive stimulation in debility; reduces excessive sweating in anxiety; helps reduce menopausal symptoms. **Warning:** Should not be taken in pregnancy.

PREPARATIONS: Infusion, tincture.

DOSE: 2–8g dried herb equivalent three times daily.

Sambucus nigra

(Caprifolicaeae)

ELDER, BLACK ELDER, PIPE TREE, HOLLUNDER, SUREAU

Elder has long and involved links with magic. It is said that witches live in the tree and their permission must be asked before any part of the plant is harvested. Burning the wood still brings the superstitious all manner of bad luck but sprigs hung in houses ward off evil witches. The symbol of sorrow and death. It is believed the crucifixion cross was fashioned from elder wood and that Judas hanged himself from an elder tree. All parts of the tree are useful and so many are their medicinal uses that it is called the people's medicine chest. A native of Europe and North Africa where is common in hedgerows and woods. A perennial shrub or small tree to 10m (33ft.) with compound leaves divided into five leaflets with serrated margins. Flowers are small, cream and massed into flat cymes 18cm (6in.) in diameter, with a strong and sweet perfume. Spring flowering is followed by clusters of deep purple to black succulent berries. Stems are filled with a soft pith. Easily cultivated.

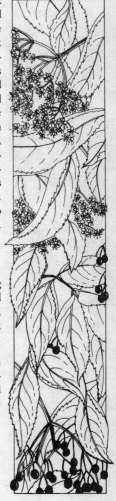

PARTS USED: Flowers, leaves, berries and bark.

ACTIVE INGREDIENTS/ACTIONS: Triterpenes, including ursolic acid; fixed oil; flavonoids including rutin and quercetin; tannins. Circulatory stimulant, astringent, diaphoretic, expectorant, anticatarrhal, anti-inflammatory; diuretic.

MEDICINAL USE: The flowers are a useful cold and flu remedy, controlling the fever and reducing catarrh production; leaves and bark are useful as a mouthwash and healer of minor burns; the berries are gently laxative when cooked but cathartic when raw.

PREPARATIONS: Infusion, decoction, tincture.

DOSE: 2-8g dried flower equivalent three times daily.

Scutellaria lateriflora

(Labiatae) also *S. galericulata and S. baicalensis*

SKULLCAP, MAD-DOG WEED, MAD WEED, HELMET FLOWER

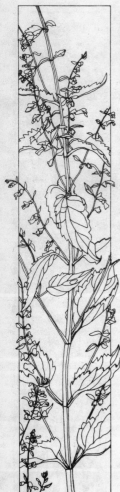

The many related species that grow around the world have found their place in traditional medicines as diverse as Native American, Chinese, Tibetan. The use is consistent. It is one of the best nervines for stressed or debilitated nervous systems. The name skullcap comes from the dried calyx which looks remarkably like a Dutch woman's bonnet. All are of similar appearance. *S. galericulata* is a perennial found near water and growing to 60cm (24in.) with square stems and opposite lanceolate leaves with serrate margins. The bright blue, lipped flowers are borne in pairs arising from the axils of the upper leaves. Flowering is in midsummer. Easily cultivated.

PARTS USED: Herb.

ACTIVE INGREDIENTS/ACTIONS: Flavonoid glycoside, scutellarin and scutellarein; flavonoids (*S. baicalensis* contains, baicalin, baicalein, wogonin, skullcap flavones); iridoids; volatile oil; tannins. Sedative, nervine, antispasmodic, anticonvulsant.

MEDICINAL USE: Calming in panic, anxiety and nervous tension; useful as a tonic in long-term depression or nervous exhaustion; helps reduce severity and frequency of fits in epilepsy.

PREPARATIONS: Infusion, tincture.

DOSE: 2-8g dried herb equivalent three times daily.

Senecio aureus

(Compositae)

LIFE ROOT, GOLDEN GROUNDSEL, SQUAW WEED

One of the most revered Native American herbs, used as a general decongestant and toning herb for the female pelvis. In Western practice, it was used initially to treat vaginal discharges but has since been found to have wider uses. Native to central United States and Canada on moist soil near water. A perennial to 60cm (24in.) with a grooved stem bearing petiolate, heart-shaped basal leaves and deeply dentate, lanceolate upper leaves. Flowers are small yellow and daisy-like in terminal corymbs, appearing in early to midsummer. Easily cultivated.

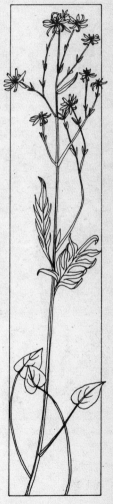

PARTS USED: Herb.

ACTIVE INGREDIENTS/ACTIONS: Pyrollizidine alkaloids, florosenine, otosenine, floridanine, senescine; sesquiterpenes. Uterine relaxant, stimulant to the gravid uterus, diuretic, mild expectorant.

MEDICINAL USE: Helps with congested pelvic conditions, including painful and excessive menstruation; symptoms of menopause; helps in functional amenorrhoea and in leucorrhoea. **Warning:** Large doses may harm the liver so should not be used except under professional advice. Should not be used in pregnancy.

PREPARATIONS: Infusion, tincture.

DOSE: For professional use only.

Smilax ornata

(Lilaceae)

SARSAPARILLA, JAMAICAN SARSAPARILLA

Used to flavour medicines and soft drinks. In the Americas and the Caribbean it has long been a favourite tonic drink after noting how the South American Indians used it as a strengthening tonic. Baldwins, the London Herbalist shop, make and sell their own sarsaparilla drinks in the shop. First used in Europe in the early sixteenth century as a cure for syphilis. Listed in European pharmacopoeias for syphilis until the twentieth century. Native to Central America and distinct from American sarsaparilla which is unrelated. A perennial creeper with a large rhizome and spreading roots. Stems are heavily thorned and bear ovate leaves with clinging tendrils in the axils. Clusters of small greenish-white flowers are borne in leaf axils. Not easily cultivated.

PARTS USED: Root.

ACTIVE INGREDIENTS/ACTIONS: Steroidal saponins including pillarin, smilasaponin and sarsaparilloside; sitosterol and stigmasterol. Alterative and anti-inflammatory, antipruritic, carminative.

MEDICINAL USE: An excellent duperative in chronic inflamed skin eruptions like eczema and psoriasis.

PREPARATIONS: Infusion, tablets, tincture.

DOSE: 2–8g dried root equivalent three times daily.

Solanum dulcamara

(Solanaceae)

BITTERSWEET, WOODY NIGHTSHADE, FELONWOOD

Not to be confused with deadly nightshade (*Atropa belladonna*) which is a different species. The name bittersweet stems from the change from bitterness to sweetness when the twigs are chewed. It has been used since the time of the ancient Greeks. Gerard said it was useful for 'those who have fallen from high places, and have therefore been bruised or beaten.' It was used to dissolve bruises and warts. The superstitious hung leaves about the necks of sheep to ward off evil spirits. Native to Europe and North America but widely distributed, especially on waste ground. A shrubby, trailing perennial with thin woody stems bearing ovate leaves, often with two basal lobes, and with entire margins. Flowers are deep violet with yellow centres in hanging cymes during mid to late summer, and are followed by red berries. Easily cultivated.

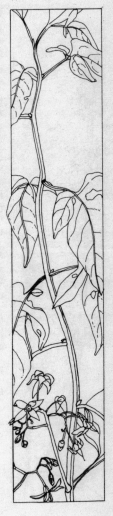

PARTS USED: 2–3–year–old stems.

ACTIVE INGREDIENTS/ACTIONS: Steroidal alkaloids, with soladulcamaridine, solanidine, solasodine, tomatidine; steroidal saponins, dulcamarin; tannin; resin. Duperative, anti–inflammatory, anti–rheumatic, stimulating expectorant, cholagogue.

MEDICINAL USE: Used in inflammatory conditions like rheumatic disease, psoriasis and eczema, especially where a sluggish liver is involved; also useful in chronic bronchitis.

PREPARATIONS: Infusion, tincture.

DOSE: 1–4g dried stem equivalent three times daily.

Stachys betonica

(Labiatae)

BETONY, WOOD BETONY, BISHOPSWORT

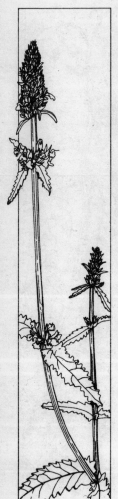

Betony has been used since ancient times and was grown in all monastery and physic gardens in Europe. Roman emperor Augustus boasted that it could cure at least 47 ailments. Since the Egyptians, it possessed additional powers to dispel evil and was worn about the body to shield 'against visions and dreams', and is reputed to be the 'most magical' plant of the Anglo-Saxons. Gerard said, 'there is a conserve made of the floures and sugar good for many things, and especially for the head ache'. Native to Europe where it grows on light sandy soils in sheltered areas. A low growing perennial herb to 50cm (20in.) high, with square stems and lanceolate, rough, leaves showing well-serrated margins. Flowers appear in midsummer as two-lipped, purple flowers with tight whorls in terminal spikes. Cultivation easy.

PARTS USED: Herb during flowering.

ACTIVE INGREDIENTS/ACTIONS: Alkaloids, including stachydrine, trigonelline and betonicine; choline; tannins. Vulnerary, astringent; circulatory tonic for head; relaxing nervine; bitter.

MEDICINAL USE: Useful in nervous or stress headaches; helpful in functional digestive upsets; useful in liver and gall-bladder disease. For wounds and bruises as a poultice.

PREPARATIONS: Infusion, tincture.

DOSE: 2–8g dried herb equivalent three times daily.

Stellaria media

(Caryophyllaceae)

CHICKWEED, STARWEED, HERBE A L'OISEAU,

A common weed around human settlement. So common that the unwise often overlook its medicinal values. Culpeper said it 'doth wonderfully temper the heat of the liver, and is effectual for all impostumes and swellings whatsoever, for all redness in the face, wheals, pushes, itch or scabs, the juice being either simply used or boiled in hog's grease'. A relished feed for birds as well as all herbivorous animals. An excellent vegetable, being either boiled as spinach or eaten as salad. Native to Europe but so widespread it is naturalized on farmed as well as wasteland especially in urban areas. A beautiful and delicate annual herb with a vigorous spreading habit and much branched, delicate stems. Leaves are small, ovate and bright pale green. Flowers appear all summer as white stars. Easily cultivated.

PARTS USED: Herb.

ACTIVE INGREDIENTS/ACTIONS: Saponins; coumarins; flavonoids; triterpenoids; carboxylic acids; vitamin C. Antipruritic, vulnerary, emollient, astringent.

MEDICINAL USE: Unsurpassable for soothing itchy and inflamed skin diseases like eczema and related dermatitis; a useful poultice in skin eruptions; taken internally in rheumatic disease.

PREPARATIONS: Poultice, creams, tincture.

DOSE: 2-8g dried herb equivalent three times daily.

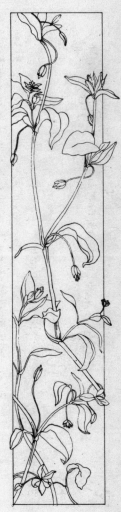

Symphytum officiale

(Boraginaceae)

COMFREY, KNITBONE, BLACKWORT, BRUISEWORT, ASS EAR

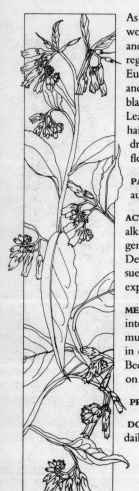

As the common names suggest, this is an ancient bone and wound healing herb. It is also an animal and human food and organic manure. The ability to stimulate bone regrowth is due to the ingredient allantoin. A native of Europe and Asia on moist to wet wasteland and meadows, and has been introduced elsewhere. A perennial on a deep, black root with erect, green, bristly stems to 1m (3ft.). Leaves are large – to 30cm (12in.) – and are succulent, hairy and decurrent. Flowers through the summer with drooping racemes of white, pink or purple, bell-shaped flowers. Easily cultivated.

PARTS USED: Herb during flowering, root harvested in autumn.

ACTIVE INGREDIENTS/ACTIONS: Allantoin; pyrollizidine alkaloids; phenolic acids, including rosmarinic, chlorogenic, caffeic; mucilage; choline; tannins; saponins. Demulcent, vulnerary, stimulant of bone, connective tissue and cartilage repair, soothing astringent, relaxing expectorant.

MEDICINAL USE: A healing agent on wounds, ulcers, internal wounds as well as bone fractures, joint sprains and muscle strains; healing in stomach ulcers and gastritis, and in colitis; used as an expectorant in bronchitis. **Warning:** Because of the pyrollizidine alkaloids take internally only on herbalist's advice.

PREPARATIONS: Infusion, decoction, creams, tincture.

DOSE: 2–8g dried herb or root equivalent three times daily.

268

Tanacetum parthenium

(Compositae)

FEVERFEW, FEATHERFEW, MIDSUMMER DAISY, FLIRTWORT, BATCHELOR'S BUTTONS

Like the elder, traditional medicine has many uses for this herb. It was used for headaches, 'women's' problems, and neuralgias. Culpeper recommended it to 'bring down women's courses speedily, and [to] help expel the dead-birth and afterbirth. For a woman to sit over hot fumes of the decoction of the herb made in water or wine. . . and in some cases, to apply the boiled herb warm to the privy parts'. It is also used as an insect repellent. Native to the south of Europe but is widely spread throughout the world. A perennial to 50cm (20in.) with a many branched stem having a mass of bright yellowish-green, slightly hairy, pinnate leaves, which look almost fern-like, and have a pungent odour. Flowers are flat, daisy-like, in clusters at the top of the plant from early summer through the summer. Easily cultivated.

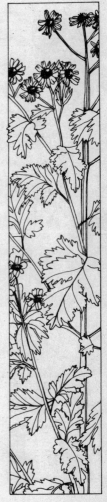

PARTS USED: Herb.

ACTIVE INGREDIENTS/ACTIONS: Volatile oil with pinene, bornyl acetate; sesquiterpene lactones, including partheno-lide; chrysanthemonin; acetylene derivatives. Febrifuge, vasodilator, analgesic, stomachic, anthelmintic, and antirheumatic.

MEDICINAL USE: Effective to treat or prevent migraine headaches where vasoconstriction is involved; in arthritis; to dysmenorrhoea; helpful after birth to restore the uterus.

PREPARATIONS: Fresh leaves, powdered leaves and tablets, tincture.

DOSE: 3–10 fresh leaves or equivalent three times daily.

Taraxacum officinale

(Compositae)

DANDELION, PIS EN LIT, LION'S TOOTH

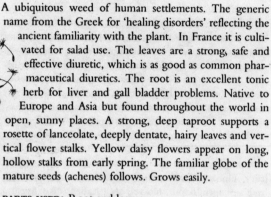

A ubiquitous weed of human settlements. The generic name from the Greek for 'healing disorders' reflecting the ancient familiarity with the plant. In France it is cultivated for salad use. The leaves are a strong, safe and effective diuretic, which is as good as common pharmaceutical diuretics. The root is an excellent tonic herb for liver and gall bladder problems. Native to Europe and Asia but found throughout the world in open, sunny places. A strong, deep taproot supports a rosette of lanceolate, deeply dentate, hairy leaves and vertical flower stalks. Yellow daisy flowers appear on long, hollow stalks from early spring. The familiar globe of the mature seeds (achenes) follows. Grows easily.

PARTS USED: Root and leaves.

ACTIVE INGREDIENTS/ACTIONS: Sesquiterpene lactones; bitter principle, taraxacin; triterpenes including taraxol, taraxerol, stigmasterol; phenolic acids; polysaccharides; carotenoids. Diuretic, tonic, antirheumatic, laxative, cholagogue.

MEDICINAL USE: The choice liver tonic; useful in inflamed gall bladder with stones; effective diuretic in raised blood pressure and water retention; useful in jaundice; gentle laxative where liver sluggishness is involved. Fresh juice is applied directly to warts.

PREPARATIONS: Fresh and dried herb; infusion, decoction of root, tincture.

DOSE: 2-12g dried herb equivalent three times daily.

Thymus vulgaris

(Labiatae) also *T. serphyllum*

GARDEN THYME, MOTHER OF THYME

Known in ancient Rome as the source of the best honey in Athens and has been used as an insecticide by burning the leaves as long as records have existed. Pliny went so far as to recommend it against all venomous creatures. The generic name comes from the Greek to fumigate. A traditional remedy for coughs, lung infections and stomach complaints. The volatile oil, thymol, has been shown to be one of the most powerful natural antiseptics. *T. serphyllum* is the wild form, and there is much natural variation in thymes. Native to the mountains of southern Europe. A creeping, aromatic perennial with thin and wiry stems bearing small, oblong, succulent leaves. Flowers appear in early summer as clusters of small, pinkish blooms among the terminal leaves of stems.

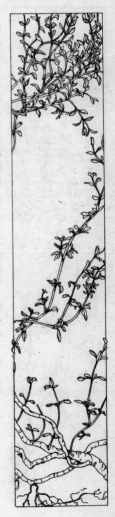

PARTS USED: Herb, collected during flowering.

ACTIVE INGREDIENTS/ACTIONS: Volatile oil with thymol, carvacrol, cineole, borneol, linalool, pinene; flavonoids including apigenin, luteolin; tannins. Antiseptic, expectorant, carminative, spasmolytic.

MEDICINAL USE: Excellent as an expectorant for whooping cough, bronchitis and congested lungs; a gargle for throat and mouth infections.

PREPARATIONS: Infusion, oil, tincture.

DOSE: 2–8g dried herb equivalent three times daily.

Tilia europaea

(Tiliaceae) also T. cordata

LIME FLOWERS, LINDEN, TILLEUL

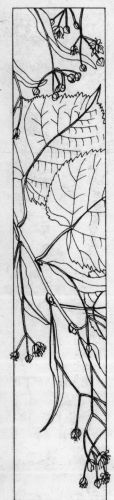

Used traditionally in Europe for colds and fevers. Recent research in the United States has shown that children with flu recovered more quickly and with fewer complications on *Tilia* tea than children given sulpho-namides or antibiotics. *Tilia* is also a relaxing herb that in France is used to help parents cope with irritable children in the afternoons after school. It is the most popular daily tisane in France. The American linden, *T. americana*, has similar uses. Native to Europe in open woodland. It is a common ornamental tree planted on footpaths and parks. A tall, deciduous tree to 35m (114ft.) with smooth bark, white wood, and toothed heart-shaped leaves. Flowers appear as hanging cymes, with sweet aroma, in spring. Easily cultivated.

PARTS USED: Flowers.

ACTIVE INGREDIENTS/ACTIONS: Volatile oil containing farnesol; flavonoids, including hesperidin, quercetin, astralagin; mucilage; tannins. Nervine, spasmolytic, hypotensive, diaphoretic.

MEDICINAL USE: Useful gentle relaxant for children and adults with anxiety, irritability; helps in nervous states affecting digestion, blood pressure, bowel function. Used in fever, colds and flu.

PREPARATIONS: Infusion, tincture.

DOSE: 2-8g dried flower equivalent three times daily.

Trifolium pratense

(Leguminosae)

RED CLOVER, PURPLE CLOVER, TREFOIL

The pink flowers are a favourite sweet snack of country children. A European meadow and pasture plant which had to be taken to North America, become naturalized, and have its medicinal properties discovered by the Native Americans before being reintroduced to Europe as a medicine. Traditionally it was used as a topical remedy for skin cancers but this has not been proven. Native to Europe but widely naturalized. A low perennial with hairy stems and trifoliate leaves with serrate margins, producing typical clover flowers coloured red to purple in the summer. Easily cultivated.

PARTS USED: Flowers.

ACTIVE INGREDIENTS/ACTIONS: Isoflavones; flavonoids; coumarins. Alterative, dermatological agent, antispasmodic, expectorant.

MEDICINAL USE: Supportive herb in treating skin disease including eczemas and psoriasis.

PREPARATIONS: Infusion, tincture.

DOSE: 2-8g dried flowers equivalent three times daily.

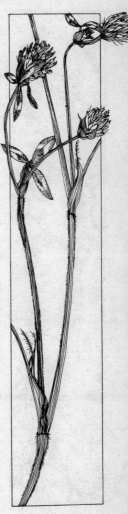

Tussilago farfara

(Compositae)

COLTSFOOT, HORSEHOOF, COUGHWORT, BULL'S FOOT

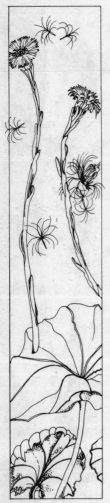

All the great ancient physicians recommended this plant as the greatest of lung medicines, especially smoked as tobacco. It is still recognized as the best herb for chesty coughs and bronchitis. The generic name, meaning cough dispeller, confirms its reputation for coughs. It was originally thought to be two different plants because the flowers appear straight from the ground in spring and have withered days or weeks before the first leaf emerges from the soil. The flowers are included in pharmacopoeias as a syrup for coughs. Native to Europe on moist wasteland but widely introduced and naturalized. A perennial with a tough, white, creeping stolons. The yellow daisy-like flowers appear on scaly stems growing to 30cm (12in.) in early spring. Large, downy, hoof-shaped leaves appear after flowering. Easily cultivated.

PARTS USED: Leaves, flowers.

ACTIVE INGREDIENTS/ACTIONS: Flavonoids, including rutin, hyperoside and isoquercetin; pyrollizidine alkaloids; mucilage; tannin. Antitussive, expectorant, demulcent, anti-inflammatory.

MEDICINAL USE: Used in dry, irritable coughing, especially with a nervous component; helps reduce bronchial spasm in asthma and bronchitis.

PREPARATIONS: Infusion, syrup, tobacco, tincture.

DOSE: 2–8g dried flower or herb equivalent three times daily.

Ulmus fulva

(Ulmaceae)

SLIPPERY ELM, RED ELM, MOOSE ELM

Native Americans had many uses for the scraped inner bark of this tree. It was a poultice for all wounds, a treatment for both constipation, because of the copious mucilage it contains, and diarrhoea because of its astringency. When it arrived in Europe it soon became a valuable convalescent food because of its copious, easily digested mucilage, which was also claimed to possess tonic and strengthening qualities. Many traditional poultices and soothing cream formulae contain *Ulmus*. Harvesting the bark kills the tree. Native to North America, found in poor soils along the east coast, this tree grows to 15m (50ft.) with rough bark and ovate leaves with serrated margins and hairs. Flowers are tiny in clusters and produce small seeds surrounded by a circular, papery 'wing'.

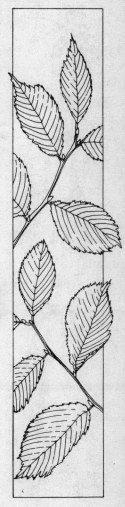

PARTS USED: Inner bark.

ACTIVE INGREDIENTS/ACTIONS: Mucilage; tannin. Demulcent, emollient, nutritive.

MEDICINAL USE: Soothes inflamed mucosae of the digestive tract; helps in pleurisy and dry bronchitic conditions; useful in debility as an easily swallowed and digested energy source; used as a poultice in boils, abscesses and infected wounds.

PREPARATIONS: Powdered bark, tablets, cream.

DOSE: 5–20g powdered bark equivalent three times daily.

Urtica dioica

(Urticaceae)

STINGING NETTLE, COMMON NETTLE

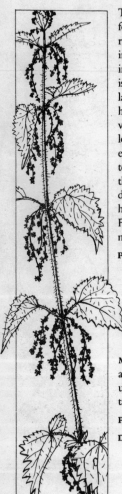

The nettle is a versatile plant. It has been used as cloth, food, dye, and medicine. The Romans used to flail their rheumatic joints with nettles to cause a warming and healing inflammation. Leaves were rubbed onto their skin during freezing British winters for warmth. The sting, which is due to ammonia in special hairs, stimulates blood circulation. *Urtica* contains both iron and the vitamin C that helps its absorption in the intestine. When leaves are harvested the stinging hairs rapidly wilt and can sting no longer. A traditional 'spring cleansing tonic' is made from equal parts of new shoots of nettle and *Galium*, which grow together. A native of Europe and Asia but naturalized throughout the world on fertile soils. The perennial form is dioecious (male and female plants) with erect stems with heart-shaped leaves bearing both plain and stinging hairs. Flowers are not striking and appear from early to late summer. Difficult to cultivate.

PARTS USED: Herb.

ACTIVE INGREDIENTS/ACTIONS: Indoles including histamine and serotonin; formic acid; acetylcholine; vitamins A and C; minerals, including iron, silica and potassium. Antihaemorrhagic, circulatory stimulant, antihistamine, dermatological agent, galactagogue, mild hypoglycaemic.

MEDICINAL USE: Fresh nettle juice is used in skin diseases and in rheumatism; it is used as an iron tonic in anaemia; used in non-insulin dependent diabetes; a support for lactating mothers.

PREPARATIONS: Juice, fresh herb, infusions, tincture.

DOSE: 2–8g dried herb equivalent three times daily.

Valeriana officinalis

(Valerianaceae)

VALERIAN, ALL–HEAL

In traditional medicine, this beautiful plant was called 'all-heal'. During World War II in Europe, it was used as a general sedative to help the civilian population cope with bombing neurosis, and as a medicine for shell-shocked soldiers. An excellent calming sedative for humans, but for cats it is exciting, producing a euphoric frenzy. The characteristic smell is loved by some people and hated by others. One traditional name is 'phu'. The smell appears only on drying the plant, especially the roots. It has been used as a spice and perfume. Native to Europe and West Asia in low-lying, damp, loamy meadows and near streams. It is naturalized in North America. A perennial with a conical rhizome and thick roots, from which a single stem rises to 80cm (31.5in.) bearing compound leaves made up of spear-like segments. Flowers appear in mid-summer as pink to white small, flattened cymes which produce tiny downy seeds to be carried on the wind. Easily cultivated.

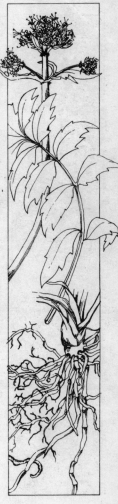

PARTS USED: Roots.

ACTIVE INGREDIENTS/ACTIONS: Volatile oil with valerinic and isovaleric acid, bornyl acetate and bornyl isovalerate; iridoids called valepotriates; alkaloids, including actinidine, valerine, valerianine and chatinine; flavonoids, tannins. Sedative, hypnotic, antispasmodic, hypotensive, mild diuretic and expectorant.

MEDICINAL USE: The most useful herb in anxiety and anxiety-based insomnia, and nervous tension; useful relaxing action on the gut in irritable bowel syndrome; applied locally for muscle spasm and cramping.

PREPARATIONS: Tablets, tincture.

DOSE: 2-15g dried root equivalent three times daily.

Viburnum opulus

(Caprifoliaceae) also *V. prunifolium*

CRAMP BARK, GUELDER ROSE, BLACK HAW, EUROPEAN CRANBERRY, WATER ELDER

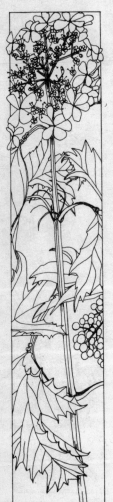

The berries make a tart-flavoured jelly and were used against scurvy. An ancient and beautiful European plant, very common in hedgerows and country lanes, which was well-known to the poet, Chaucer, who advised that one should 'picke the berries hen right as they grow and ete hem in'. The European (*V. opulus*) and the American (*prunifolium*) species have similar constituents and uses. *V. opulus* is native to Europe, North Africa and West Asia but widely introduced. It is a small shrub with lobed leaves and clusters of small white flowers in midsummer, followed by bunches of red and scarlet berries which are edible. Easily cultivated.

PREPARATIONS: Bark.

ACTIVE INGREDIENTS/ACTIONS: Hydroquinnones, including arbutin and hydroquinone; coumarins, including scopoletin and scopoline; tannins. Antispasmodic to smooth and skeletal muscle, sedative, astringent.

MEDICINAL USE: Used in spasmodic pain of periods, and in general muscle cramping, especially in the intestine; a uterine relaxant in threatened miscarriage.

PREPARATIONS: Decoction, tincture.

DOSE: 2-8g dried bark equivalent three times daily.

Vinca major

(Apocynaceae) also *V. minor*

GREATER PERIWINKLE

Possibly used as an early contraceptive, it was said that *Vinca* could induce love between man and wife if it were eaten in a mixture of earthworms and houseleek. No doubt without any connection with the above, it was also associated with death and placed on the coffins of children. The plant is the subject of recent pharmaceutical interest. The related *V. rosea* is the source of two pharmaceutical drugs used against leukaemias, vincristine and vinblastine. A native of Europe on alkaline soils. The five-petalled flowers are the striking feature of this perennial creeper with glossy, ovate leaves having a lighter green stripe down their centres. Flowers appear in the leaf axils in early summer but are not followed by any fruit. Easily cultivated.

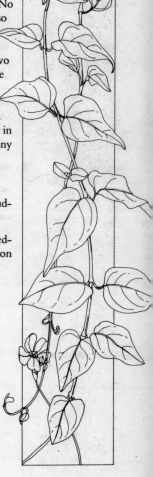

PARTS USED: Herb.

ACTIVE INGREDIENTS/ACTIONS: Indole alkaloids, including reserpine; tannins. Anti-haemorrhagic, astringent.

MEDICINAL USE: An astringent in excess menstrual bleeding and vaginal discharges; used in nosebleeds and on haemorrhoids.

PREPARATIONS: Infusion, tincture.

DOSE: 2-8g dried herb equivalent three times daily.

Viola tricolor

(Violaceae)

HEARTSEASE, WILD PANSY, LOVE–LIES–BLEEDING; KISS–HER–IN–THE–BUTTERY

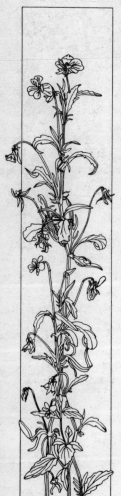

Many herbs were associated with the powers of love charms. This herb was recommended for mending broken hearts (but not for heart disease). An ancient traditional remedy for skin inflammations and 'against scabs and itchings of the whole body.' A native of Europe, especially on waste ground or following cultivation of any soil or garden. Naturalized in North America. Short annual or biennial herb with fragile stems and lanceolate, dentate leaves. Yellow, white and purple flowers in the classic pansy shape. Flowering is throughout the summer. Easily cultivated.

PARTS USED: Herb.

ACTIVE INGREDIENTS/ACTIONS: Flavonoids; saponin; methyl salycilate; resin; tannin. Anti-inflammatory, diuretic, antirheumatic, expectorant.

MEDICINAL USE: A common herb in prescriptions for skin disease especially eczema, for rheumatism and gout.

PREPARATIONS: Infusion, tincture.

DOSE: 2–8g dried herb equivalent three times daily.

Viscum album

(Loranthaceae)

MISTLETOE

A large and distinctive parasitic plant. There are strong magical associations, which still survive in the custom of hanging it in houses at Christmas. It was sacred to the ancient Druids, and sprigs were carried to dispel evil spirits. The Latin name *Viscum* refers to the stickiness of the seeds, which allows the seeds to stick to the new host tree's branches and germinate. Native to Europe. Leaves of this evergreen are light green, leathery and oar-shaped. Tiny flowers appear in threes within leaf axils during early summer, and produce the pale green to white, semi-translucent berries which ripen in late autumn. Difficult to cultivate.

PARTS USED: Leaves, berries.

ACTIVE INGREDIENTS/ACTIONS: Glycoproteins; viscotoxins; phenolic acids; flavonoids; lignans. Vasodilator, hypotensive, sedative, reputedly antineoplastic.

MEDICINAL USE: Used for certain types of high blood pressure, especially with arterial disease and when nervous conditions are present. **Warning:** Should not be taken except under professional supervision.

PREPARATIONS: Decoction, tincture.

DOSE: 2–8g dried herb or berry equivalent three times daily.

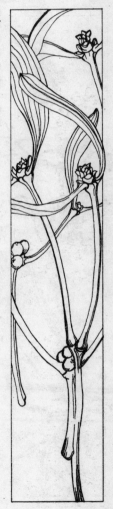

Vitex agnus-castus

(Verbenaceae)

CHASTEBERRY, AGNUS CASTUS, MONK'S PEPPER

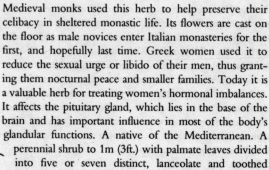

Medieval monks used this herb to help preserve their celibacy in sheltered monastic life. Its flowers are cast on the floor as male novices enter Italian monasteries for the first, and hopefully last time. Greek women used it to reduce the sexual urge or libido of their men, thus granting them nocturnal peace and smaller families. Today it is a valuable herb for treating women's hormonal imbalances. It affects the pituitary gland, which lies in the base of the brain and has important influence in most of the body's glandular functions. A native of the Mediterranean. A perennial shrub to 1m (3ft.) with palmate leaves divided into five or seven distinct, lanceolate and toothed leaflets. Small, purple flowers appear in spike-like cymes in the summer. The whole plant is strongly aromatic. Small seeds are produced. Cultivated with care.

PARTS USED: Seeds.

ACTIVE INGREDIENTS/ACTIONS: Volatile oils; flavonoids; glycoside; bitter, casteine. Hormonal, acting on the pituitary gland.

MEDICINAL USE: Used in premenstrual syndrome, excessive menstrual flow, menopause.

PREPARATIONS: Infusion, tincture.

DOSE: 2–8g dried berries equivalent three times daily.

Zanthoxylum americanum

(Rutaceae)

PRICKLY ASH, TOOTHBRUSH BUSH

Native Americans introduced the white settlers to this cure for toothache. The pain of nineteenth-century dentistry made any alternative cure for toothache worth its weight in gold and *Zanthoxylum* soon crossed the Atlantic to a great welcome. It is now recognized as a general circulatory stimulant with wide application in natural medicine. Native to the United States on rich woodland soil. A shrub with palmate leaves having stiff lanceolate leaflets and sharp spines on the branches. Flowers appear in early spring in leaf axils. Can be cultivated.

PARTS USED: Bark and berries.

ACTIVE INGREDIENTS/ACTIONS: Coumarins; alkaloids, including chelerythrine, magnoflorine, nitidine; resin, tannins, volatile oil. Circulatory stimulant, local counter irritant; diaphoretic, antirheumatic, sialagogue.

MEDICINAL USE: Used in peripheral circulatory conditions such as varicose eczema or chilblains; in skin, joint and general inflammatory disorders where sluggish circulation is a factor; useful in debilitated digestion with colic and flatulence.

PREPARATIONS: Decoction, tincture.

DOSE: 2–8g dried bark equivalent three times daily.

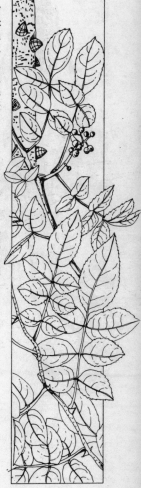

Zea mays

(Graminae)

CORNSILK, MAIZE

Maize or corn is a valuable cereal food for humans and animals. The kernels contain starch, an oil low in saturated fatty acids while rich in the polyunsaturated type that lowers the risks of circulation and heart disease. The kernel coat passes through the intestine undigested and thus provides a useful measure of the time taken for digested food to pass through the intestine. The silks, which are not usually eaten or used by humans, are a urinary system herb. Native to South America, but now cultivated throughout the world. An annual grass with male and female flowers on each plant. The male tassel sits on top of the plant while the one to three female flowers sit in leaf axils and produce hair-like stigmas to catch pollen dropped from the male flowers. As soon as the ovaries in the cob are fertilized, the stigmas dry to a rusty brown and the yellow kernels develop. Easily cultivated.

PARTS USED: Stigmas and styles.

ACTIVE INGREDIENTS/ACTIONS: Saponins; allantoin; sterols, sitosterol, stigmasterol; alkaloid, hordenine; tannins. Diuretic, demulcent.

MEDICINAL USE: Soothing for an inflamed urinary tract from kidney to penis or urethral opening, especially for cystitis, urethritis, bladder infections, nephritis. Useful in urinary stones or calculi.

PREPARATIONS: Infusion, tincture.

DOSE: 2–12g dried silks equivalent three times daily.

Zingiber officinalis

(Zingiberaceae)

GINGER

An important example of a popular culinary spice that was first used as a medicine. The ancient Greeks and Chinese used ginger as medicine not as food. When the Romans invaded Britain in AD 43 they had ginger in their medicinal kits. The crystallized roots are a prized confection around the world. Native to south-east Asia, but introduced worldwide, and via Spain to the tropics where it is now grown commercially. The best quality ginger still comes from Asia. A perennial with a thick tuberous root sending up thin, reed-like stems with long tapering leaves and purplish flowers in spikes. Roots are harvested after leaves have died in the autumn. Easily cultivated.

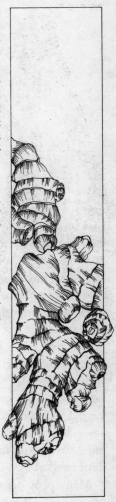

PARTS USED: Root.

ACTIVE INGREDIENTS/ACTIONS: Volatile oil with cineole, borneol, linalool, zingiberol, camphene, citral; phenols including gingerols, gingerdiols and shogoals. Peripheral circulatory stimulant, carminative, anti-emetic, diaphoretic, hypocholesterolaemic.

MEDICINAL USE: Used for poor peripheral circulation with Raynaud's disease or chilblains, and as a warming circulatory stimulant in lung infections; in travel sickness; useful in dyspepsia and flatulence.

PREPARATIONS: Fresh root, infusion, tincture.

DOSE: 2-8g dried root equivalent three times daily.

CHAPTER SEVEN
Home Remedies

EXPLORING HOME REMEDIES IS RE-CREATING THE MOST ANCIENT use of herbs. Households had to decide the nature of their illnesses, decide on the best remedy, go out to collect the herbs and prepare their own medicines in the kitchen. The herbs collected had to be chosen from those that grew in the locality. Occasionally efficient herbs were imported from neighbouring localities or from other countries. The gift of myrrh that was brought to the infant Christ is perhaps the best known example of an excellent herbal medicine brought from afar.

Most herbs are seasonal and had to be harvested at the best time and stored until, or in case, they were needed at other times of the year. This led to skill in choosing the best time of year, month and even day to harvest to retain the highest concentration of active ingredients. Skill in storing herbs keeps their healing potency alive until needed.

Many people continue to grow or harvest their own herbs for use at home. However, even those without green fingers or the confidence to identify and collect their own supplies from the countryside can be skilful home healers. All useful herbs for a home-remedy kit can be bought from reliable suppliers in most large cities of most countries. Using herbs at home also provides safe, effective, practical, and cheap medicines.

Safe use of home remedies is assured by using only herbs that are recommended and never collecting or growing your own herbs unless you are certain of their identification. Always stick to recommended doses.

There are thousands of herbs that have been used as medicines. Many are effective but as many are probably less so and not worth using, especially when there are well-recommended alternatives. There are also a larger number of books, booklets and magazine articles recommending herbs for this or that use. Often advice is either medically unsound or the suggested herbal useless. It is always best to check both the medical and herbal qualifications of the person giving the advice. There is a list of books by qualified herbalists on pages 310-11.

Self-diagnosis and medication can be safe if simple rules are followed. Over 90 per cent of all illnesses taken to doctors are simple conditions that can be treated at home. There is already a large market for 'over the counter remedies' for most illnesses in the medical dictionary. Coughs, colds, indigestion, mouth ulcers, colic, constipation, headaches, 'rheumatism', muscular aches and pains, nervousness, insomnia, chilblains, insect stings, varicose veins, nappy rash, eczema and so on. All these can be treated effectively with herbs.

It is essential that the diagnosis is correct. If there is any doubt, check with a doctor or medical herbalist. Once the diagnosis is confirmed, it may still be possible to treat with both herbs and confidence. Take diagnosis very seriously. The wrong diagnosis may result in choosing the wrong herbal remedy. But it can also be dangerous. An incorrect diagnosis may mean neglecting a serious condition that needs urgent treatment. Any delay in seeking essential treatment could bring serious consequences.

Simple symptoms can be due to serious illness. Stomach pain or headaches are common and usually have simple causes like indigestion or a little nervous tension. To be safe, even when you feel your own diagnosis is correct, always report to a doctor or medical herbalist any diarrhoea, pain in the abdomen, chest or head, or any dizzy spells that last three days or more.

HOME-REMEDY KIT

Whatever a home is, it is not a pharmacy. All possible herbs cannot be grown or stored ready for any need. This would be too impractical but also unnecessary. Like a portable first-aid box, the contents of the herbal home-remedy kit are the bare minimum for most conditions that are either likely to occur at home or can be treated safely and effectively at home. There is no best or perfect number or choice of herbs to include. Any herbalist or experienced user of herbs will have their own selection.

Below I suggest a good starter kit. It is based on long experience with teaching herbal medicine and with listening to students and patients who have used herbs at home. The kit is assembled with the following criteria in mind:

- a small number of effective herbs, which are:

- safe to use

- simple to prepare and administer

- found in most kitchens, gardens, local parks, or bought easily

- covers the most common ailments that can be self-treated safely

The number of herbs is kept to thirty, for no particular reason. Note by looking herbs up in the Materia Medica that each herb has several actions. This explains how most of the herbs in the kit can treat different conditions. There is nothing sacrosanct about this list. You can replace herbs or add others as your experience grows or according to what you wish or need to treat. Do experiment but always work with reliable reference books or qualified herbalists.

HERBS FOR THE HOME-REMEDY KIT

HERB	USES	FORM USED
Agrimony *Agrimonia eupatoria*	mild diarrhoea, indigestion, sore throats, cystitis	infusion
Arnica *Arnica montana*	bruises, sprains	tincture, cream
Calendula *Calendula officinalis*	cuts, stings, rashes, burns, thrush, athlete's foot	tincture, infusion, cream
Chamomile *Matricaria recutita*	digestion, rashes, burns, restlessness, teething	infusion, cream
Clove oil *Syzygium aromaticum*	toothache	oil
Comfrey *Symphytum officinale*	sprains, wounds, psoriasis	fresh leaf poultice, cream
Cramp bark *Viburnum opulus*	period pains, muscle cramp or spasm	decoction, tincture, creams
Dandelion *Taraxacum officinale*	water retention, digestion, warts	infusion, sap (warts)
Elder flower *Sambucus nigra*	Hay fever, catarrh, colds, flu	infusion

HERB	USES	FORM USED
Eucalyptus *Eucalyptus* spp.	wounds, colds, flu, sinusitis	oil, inhalation
Fennel *Foeniculum vulgare*	digestion, flatulence, colic	seeds, infusion
Feverfew *Tanacetum parthenium*	migraine, rheumatic pain	fresh or dried leaf, tincture
Figs *Ficus carica*	mild laxative	fruit, syrup
Garlic *Allium sativum*	antiseptic, catarrh, lung infections, food poisoning, worms, warts	whole cloves, pearls, tablets
Ginger *Zingiber officinalis*	chilblains, cold hands and feet, travel sickness, morning sickness.	fresh or powdered root, infusion
Lavender *Lavandula officinalis*	antiseptic, wounds, stings, bites, muscle spasm, relaxant	oil
Lemon balm *Melissa officinalis*	restlessness, insomnia	fresh or frozen herb infusion
Lime flower *Tilia europea*	flu, fevers, relaxant, restless children, insomnia	infusion
Linseed *Linum usitatissimum*	constipation, boils, gastritis	crushed seed
Liquorice *Glycyrrhiza glabra*	sore throats, gastritis, arthritis and eczema, flavouring medicines	dried root, decoctions, solid extract

HOME REMEDIES

HERB	USES	FORM USED
Marshmallow *Althaea officinalis*	boils, splinters, sore throats, oesophagitis	decoction, poultice
Meadowsweet *Filipendula ulmaria*	indigestion, excess acidity, colitis	infusion
Mint *Mentha* spp.	digestion, flatulence, colic	infusion
Myrrh *Commiphora molmol*	cuts, wounds; mouth-wash for sore throats and mouth ulcers	tincture
Oak bark (powder) *Quercus robur*	bleeding or weeping wounds, mouth ulcers, gingivitis	decoction, powder
Ribwort *Plantago lanceolata*	bleeding wounds, sore throats, catarrh	infusion
St John's wort *Hypericum perforatum*	burns, earache, sciatica, wounds, menstrual pain	infusion, infused oil
Thyme *Thymus vulgaris*	colds, congested chests, respiratory infections, worms	tincture, infusion
Valerian *Valeriana officinalis*	anxiety, insomnia, muscle spasm	decoction, tincture
Yarrow *Achillea millefolium*	nosebleeds, fever management	bruised leaf, infusion

There are no 'one and only' remedies for most common ailments but the following table lists tried and trusted remedies that are easy to apply and safer to use.

AILMENTS AND HELPFUL HOME REMEDIES

AILMENT	HOME REMEDIES
Antiseptic	Washes with infusions of *Calendula*, lotions of myrrh or lavender oil diluted in water, or cut fresh garlic rubbed onto the affected part. Fresh garlic disinfects the stomach.
Bites/stings	Dab lavender oil or *Calendula* tincture on neat.
Boils/spots	Poultice of marshmallow or linseed will draw out a boil and neat oil of lavender or tincture of *Calendula* helps heal and protect.
Bleeding grazes or wounds	Sprinkling of oak bark or applying a poultice of ribwort leaf helps stop bleeding. *Calendula* tincture and lavender or eucalyptus oil will keep germ-free.
Bruises/sprains	*Arnica* or comfrey cream applied regularly, or wrap a freshly crushed comfrey leaf around the part daily.
Burns	First degree burns where the skin is red and slightly blistered heal with St John's wort infused oil or washing with infusions of *Calendula* or chamomile. Let dry or wrap in crushed fresh comfrey leaf.
Catarrh	Infusions of elder flower, liquorice, and ribwort if not infected, otherwise include thyme and eat garlic.
Chilblains	Ginger root infusion warms the peripheral areas.
Colds	Eat garlic or drink thyme infusions to kill bacteria; take elder flower and lime flower teas to manage the fever which helps kill the virus. (See sore throats.)
Cold sores	Apply neat lavender or lemon balm oil, or tincture of *Calendula*.

AILMENT	HOME REMEDIES
Cystitis	Agrimony, thyme and marshmallow infusion regularly.
Colic	See digestion. Children and babies' colic can be relieved with half-strength chamomile, meadowsweet, agrimony or peppermint tea.
Diarrhoea	Treat only mild diarrhoeas. Use garlic or thyme if due to food poisoning and strong black tea, agrimony or decoctions of oak bark to stop the diarrhoea.
Digestion (poor or sluggish)	Dandelion root decoction or leaf infusion or salad to stimulate, but infusions of chamomile, mint, ginger, or fennel to calm.
Earache/ear boils	Infused oil of St John's wort, 3–4 drops twice daily.
Fevers (mild)	Controlled, not stopped, with infusions of elder flower and lime flower.
Flatulence	Fennel seeds chewed; infusions of chamomile, mint or ginger.
Flu	See colds.
Food poisoning	Mild forms solved by eating 3–5 cloves garlic daily or infusion of thyme.
Gastritis	Meadowsweet, chamomile or agrimony infusion, with liquorice root.
Gingivitis	Oak bark powder made into thin paste as mouthwash or myrrh tincture diluted 1 to 10 with water as mouthwash.
Hay fever	Start 2 months before season with elder flower and ribwort infusion daily.

AILMENT	HOME REMEDIES
Headache	Migraines often stopped or prevented with 3-5 fresh or dried leaves of feverfew daily; nervous headache eased by relaxing with lemon balm or lime flower infusions.
Indigestion	Meadowsweet or agrimony infusion.
Insomnia	Cause must be found but mild anxious forms eased with lime flower, valerian, or lemon balm infusions before bed and no caffeine drinks after midday. Sitting in a warm bath with10-15 drops of lavender oil before bed very successful.
Morning sickness	Infusion of chamomile, ginger or mint.
Mouth ulcers	Tincture of myrrh applied neat or used as a mouth-wash diluted 1 to 10 in water. Oak bark mouth-wash.
Muscle spasms	Lavender oil, 1 teaspoon in an egg cup of house-hold vegetable oil and gently massaged into the affected parts. Valerian or cramp bark internally helps.
Nosebleeds	Carefully insert a bruised leaf of yarrow into the bleeding nostril with the leaf protruding. Pinch nostrils together for 10 minutes.
Period pains	Tincture or decoction of cramp bark. Add valerian if a nervous or anxiety component.
Piles	Cream of oak bark and marigold.
Psoriasis	Comfrey and marigold cream.
Rashes	Infusions or compresses of chamomile or marigold for irritations like eczema, seborrhoea, nappy rash; marigold tincture neat on fungal rashes. Liquorice helps the metabolism.

AILMENT	HOME REMEDIES
Respiratory infections	Thyme infusions, or garlic cloves. See sore throats.
Restless children	Infusion of lime flower, lemon balm, or chamomile. Valerian if hysterical.
Relaxation	Infusion of lemon balm, lime flower, chamomile, or valerian.
Rheumatic pain	Feverfew as fresh leaf or tincture for pain; dandelion root decoction to help elimination processes. Liquorice for the metabolic processes.
Sinusitis	Steam inhalation with thyme and eucalyptus oils.
Sore throats	Gargle with 1 part myrrh tincture diluted in 10 of water; painful throat soothed with sipping strong infusion of marshmallow, agrimony or liquorice.
Splinters	A poultice of marshmallow leaf or linseed will draw them out.
Thrush	Infusion or tincture of marigold as wash on general body and as douche for vaginal thrush.
Travel sickness	Chew eighth of an inch slice fresh ginger root 20 minutes before travel and then during travel.
Teething pain	Infusion of chamomile.
Toothache	One or two drops of clove oil on the culprit.
Warts	Apply fresh dandelion latex or garlic juice daily for 2-3 weeks.
Water retention	Infusion of dandelion leaf.
Worms	Infusion of thyme or fresh garlic cloves.

PREPARATIONS

Herbalists use as many different preparations to deliver their drugs to the affected parts as do doctors. The most common internal forms of medicine are tinctures and infusions, which are extracts of herbs in alcohol or water respectively. Herbalists tend to combine a number of herbs in a prescription rather than using a 'simple', which is a single herb in a medicine. It is easy to mix tinctures or combine different amounts of dry herb to make a liquid medicine or 'tea' mix for a patient. Both the combinations of herbs and the proportions of each can be varied endlessly this way. Pills and tablets are fixed in composition and only the dose can be varied.

Creams and ointments are also used regularly to apply herbs on or just under the skin. But pills, tablets, powders, pessaries, suppositories, lotions, linctuses, syrups, compresses and poultices are also widely used. Apart from creams and ointments, most of these other forms of medicine are too complicated to make at home. The simple preparations recommended in the ailment table (above) are quite efficient for most home applications.

INFUSIONS AND DECOCTIONS

These are important but are often confused. An infusion is steeping or 'brewing' dried or fresh herb in boiling water. A decoction is simmering plant roots, bark or seeds in boiling water for at least ten minutes.

The cup of tea that the British have with breakfast, often with milk and sugar, is an infusion. (This tea is also a herbal remedy useful as a diuretic and stimulant, but that is a separate matter.) Herbal infusions are also made with water but, unlike the drink of tea which is 'brewed' for *not more than three minutes*, they should be allowed to stand for ten to fifteen minutes at least. The longer the better. It is useful to make a whole day's requirements of infusion in one batch, either in the morning or the evening before, straining off the required dose three or four times a day as required. Fresh or dried herbaceous material (leaves, flowers, finely chopped soft roots) can be infused. Infusions extract water soluble components of plants like mucilage, tannins, saponins and flavonoids. They do not extract fixed oils, resins, or alkaloids, which require a mixture of alcohol and water to dissolve them.

Herbal infusions are made with 1oz (30g) dried herb to 1 pint of boiling water. Fresh plant material can be used but remember that it is usually 80-90 per cent water so four to five times as much is needed. Always use a teapot or jug with a good lid or a thermos flask to keep any volatile oils from being lost. Use the same proportions in making a decoction but soak the dried roots or bark in the water for twelve hours before bringing to the boil and simmering. Allow to stand for as long as possible, strain and drink. Both infusions and decoctions will keep for forty-eight hours in a refrigerator, but are best made daily. The usual dosage for adults is one cup or small mug three times a day. For children older than ten years, use half the adult dose and for infants (three to ten years) use a quarter.

CREAMS

Creams are water-based medications designed to soak into the skin so the medication can be carried deep into the skin from where it can be absorbed. Creams are useful for applying medicine to affected skin or to structures just below the surface (joints, veins etc.). Sometimes the medicine is needed on the skin (eczema) and at others it is so the medication can be absorbed through to skin to reach affected parts like joints. Creams are also soothing to the skin.

Marigold (herbal as well as homoeopathic) can be bought but it is easy to make your own. The simplest way is to use emulsifying ointment BP (British Pharmacopoeia), which can be bought in good chemists. Make a double strength infusion of the chosen herb or a mixture (for example, chamomile, marigold and com-frey). Take 50g (2oz) of emulsifying ointment and heat it gently in a double boiler (or over a water bath) until it melts. Add 25ml (5 teaspoons) of the still-warm infusion. Take the mixture from the heat, stand it in a cold water bath and stir gently until it starts to thicken. Add 5 drops of friar's balsam (to preserve the cream). Pour or spoon the cream into small jars and seal. *Label straight away before you forget the herb used, and date the batch.* Make small batches each time unless you have an army to treat. A little cream goes a long way and lasts a long time.

INFUSED OIL

An infused oil is a way of extracting the medicinal value of a herb into an oil which can then be applied directly to the skin or used to make thicker ointments. Oils and ointments are usually used where a degree of skin protection is required.

St John's wort oil is simple to make. Harvest enough of the yel-low flowers during the summer to fill a 450 or 900g (1 or 2lb) screw-cap jam jar. Pour over the fresh flowers enough sunflower or maize (corn) oil to fill the jar. Place the jar in a sunny spot for four to six weeks. The oil turns a deep red and the constituents of the flowers diffuse out into the oil. Decant the oil into a clean dark jar for use. Infused oils of other plants, like comfrey, can be made by heating chopped herb in the oil over a water bath for six hours, then pressing out the oil and filtering it.

Useful comfrey-infused oil can be made. Harvest about 1kg (2.25lb) comfrey leaf in midsummer, just as the plant starts flow-ering. Chop coarsely and place in a large saucepan. Add 2l (3.33pt) of light vegetable oil (rapeseed, sunflower or maize) and bring gently to the boil. When the streams of tiny bubbles stop, the water in the leaf has been boiled out. Remove from the heat, cover and leave to infuse for twenty-four hours. Strain and bottle in dark con-tainers filled to the top to reduce oxidation during storage.

OINTMENT

Simple ointments can be made from infused oils. Weigh a quantity of oil before placing it in a pan over a water bath. Heat the oil. Weigh out a sheet of beeswax to 10 per cent of the weight of the oil. Tear the wax sheet into small pieces and add to the hot infused oil. Stir until dissolved. Pour into small jars. Put lids on jars and allow to cool and set. Label immediately with herb ingredients and date, before you forget.

POULTICE

This is a useful way of applying herbs to the skin. They are usually applied hot which increases the blood flow to the area and encourages uptake of the herbs as well as healing action. A poultice of marshmallow or pulverized linseed is useful on boils or splinters. Take 1 dessertspoon of dried herb and moisten with boiling water. When cooled to a tolerable temperature place over the boil or splinter and hold in place by tying a muslin bandage over the herb. Leave for one hour then repeat.

DRYING HERBS

Many of the herbs in the home-remedy kit grow in gardens, parks or in the countryside where productive and healthy walks can be organized. Drying herbs preserves their medicinal value at their peak, and means the herb is always available. A few simple rules will help you have the best quality dried herbs:

- Always make sure you know which species of plant is used and that you can identify it.
- Harvest the right part/s of the plant and harvest them at the best time of year for the active ingredients. Most leaves and

flowering parts are best collected early during the flowering period. Harvest when any dew or rain has dried and preferably before the heat of the midday sun. Roots, barks, and fruits are best harvested in the autumn.

- Dry the herbs carefully by spreading them out in a thin layer on paper in a warm (not hot), well-aerated room or cupboard. Keep herbs out of direct sun. Drying in darkness preserves the colour. Roots should be washed and cut into quarter-inch pieces before they are dried.
- When dried, herbs should be stored in paper bags in a dry, cool, dark room.
- Make sure every herb is carefully labelled with name and harvest date. It is remarkable how similar many plants look when they are dried.

CHAPTER EIGHT
Growing Herbs

GROWING HERBS IS AN ANCIENT PRACTICE. LONG BEFORE ornamental gardening, for either decoration or pleasure, monasteries were cultivating herb gardens. Growing herbs is an obvious solution to the inconvenience of wandering to collect them from the countryside. Since most medicinal herbs are also beautiful plants in their own right, the medicinal garden easily became an attractive display. It is no surprise that the landed wealthy families of sixteenth-century Europe had elaborately patterned herb gardens arranged to be as visible to their house guests as their indoor art treasures.

Medicinal herbs can be grown wherever there is space for a garden. The great number of plants to choose from offers enormous variety of shape, form, colour and habit. As with growing any plants, care must be taken to match the choice of plants to the available soil type, space and aspect. There is no point trying to grow African desert plants in the outdoors of northern Europe, or attempting to cultivate the soft and delicate temperate forest floor plants in the heat of a Mediterranean summer. Wherever in the world a herb garden is planned there will be local medicinal plants to consider and a large range of imported plants suitable to the environment.

Growing medicinal plants means additional considerations. If the garden is planned purely for ornament, the space allocated to each species and its arrangement is left to the physical and decorative constraints. However, if the garden is to be a 'working' garden, harvests must be considered.

Herbs that are harvested daily for food or infusions should be planted so they are easily accessible from paths. Herbs that are to be harvested when mature for use throughout the year must be in sufficient quantity to meet needs. This requires that both a sufficient area be planted for each herb and that allowance be made for the potentially large gaps after harvest. Annuals like chamomile are harvested during flowering in late summer and large amounts are needed for a typical household's annual use. Even more space may have to be allocated for *Calendula* whose flower heads are harvested throughout the summer and autumn, but again large amounts are needed. For such plants, it may be better to consider growing them in special beds where rows can be planted as in a vegetable plot.

Don't forget that many useful medicinal 'herbs' are large shrubs or trees. This is not of special importance where they are grown for interest, but harvesting the bark and roots of trees drastically changes their shape if it doesn't kill them.

Many useful herbs can be grown in lawns (*Taraxacum, Plantago*) or among other plants, almost as companion plants. *Convallaria, Geranium* spp., and *Stellaria* grow happily in the cool shaded spaces below trees or shrubs.

Pots and other containers are particularly useful for medicinal herbs. Attractive shapes and colours can be grown near the house for enjoyment and easy harvest. The containers can also be replaced with freshly planted ones as they are harvested or go past their best. Don't fall into the common trap with pots and containers, namely ignoring the soil type and physical needs of the plants. Too many pots of thyme or rosemary fail because they are grown in humus rich soils and are over-watered. Always investigate the native habitat of plants or look up the recommendations on seed packets or nursery labels.

Indoor herbs are possible but the usual restriction applies. Indoors is a dark environment unless sunny windows or special lighting are available. It is unlikely that there will be enough space to grow sufficient quantities on the average window-sill. But small pots can be rotated from outside stock, ensuring both a warming display and a convenient supply. Stick to herbs that are used in small quantities at a time (basil, chives, *Mentha* spp., *Tanacetum*).

Many wild plants are interesting and valuable herbal medicines. Do not dig up wild plants, except from your own land or with the permission of the landowner. However, small quantities of seeds can be collected for home propagation. Make sure the seeds are mature when collected, dry carefully before storing somewhere very cool, dark and dry until planting time.

Growing wild plants from seeds is often a challenging and humbling experience. Wild plants are not always rampant weeds that would grow on a sheet of glass. Many are perfectly evolved to specific niches in the ecosystem and, unless these can be carefully duplicated at home, failure is inevitable. Many seeds contain complicated dormancy mechanisms, which will frustrate all efforts at germination until the correct key is placed in the lock. Some wild plants grow only in close physical contact with other plants with which they have either a parasitic or commensal relationship.

Plants, both wild and domesticated, can also be propagated from cuttings, layering, splitting clumps or bulbs, tubers, etc. This is an economical way of multiplying plants at home and increasing your collection. Avoid disappointment by researching the best way of propagating each species.

The following table gives basic guidelines for growing many popular and useful medicinal herbs in household gardens of any size.

PLANT	TYPE	HEIGHT	SOIL	POSITION	PROPOGA-TION
Achillea millifolium	P	50cm	light, drained	sunny	seeds
Agrimonia	P	50cm	light, drained	sunny	seeds
Alchemilla	P	30cm	drained	sunny	seeds, division
Allium	P	30cm	light, rich	sunny	seeds, bulbs
Aloysia	P	60cm	rich, drained	sunny	seeds, cuttings
Althaea	P	1m	medium, damp, rich	sun, semi-shade	seeds
Armoracia	P	1m	medium, heavy	sunny	root division
Arnica	P	50cm	light, rich	sunny	root division
Artemesia	P	1.5m	medium, heavy	sunny	seeds
Calendula	A	50cm	light-medium	sunny	seeds
Cardus	A	1m	medium-heavy, rich	sunny	seeds
Centaurea	A	30cm	light, drained	sunny	seeds
Convallaria	P	20cm	medium-heavy	semi-shade	bulbs
Coriandum	A	50cm	light-medium	sunny	seeds
Digitalis	Bi	1.5m	rich, drained	shade-sunny	seeds
Filipendula	P	1.5m	medium, rich, damp	sunny	seeds, root division
Foeniculum	P	1.5m	rich, drained	sunny	seeds
Gaultheria	P	20cm	rich	shade	seeds, cuttings
Gentiana	P	1m	deep, rich	semi-shade	seeds, root division
Glechoma	P	10cm	light, drained	semi-shade	seeds

P = perennial   A = annual   Bi = biennial

GROWING HERBS

PLANT	TYPE	HEIGHT	SOIL	POSITION	PROPOGA-TION
Glycyrrhiza	P	1m	light, drained	sunny	root division
Hamamelis	P	4–5m	light, rich	sunny	seeds, layering
Humulus	A	to 5m	medium, rich	sunny	seeds, root division
Hyssopus	P	20cm	light	sunny	seeds
Inula	P	2m	medium-heavy	sun	root division
Lavandula	P	1m	light-medium	sunny	cuttings
Marrubrium	P	50cm	light-heavy	sunny	seeds, root division
Matricaria	A	30cm	medium	sunny	seeds
Melilotus	Bi	30cm	medium	semi-shade	seeds
Melissa	P	1m	light, rich	sunny	root division
Mentha	P	50cm	medium, rich	sunny	cuttings
Nepeta	P	50cm	light-medium	sun-shade	cuttings
Ocimum	P	50cm	light, drained	sunny	seeds
Origanum	P	60cm	light, drained	sunny	seeds, division
Petroselinum	Bi	30cm	light, rich	sunny	seeds
Rosemarinus	P	1m	light-medium	sunny	cuttings
Salvia	P	1m	light, rich	sunny	cuttings, seeds
Sambucus	P	5m	medium-heavy	sunny	seeds
Sanguinaria	P	40cm	light, rich	shady	cuttings
Saponaria	P	50cm	light, rich	sun-shade	root division
Stachys	P	60cm	light-medium	sunny	seeds

P = perennial   A = annual   Bi = biennial

PLANT	TYPE	HEIGHT	SOIL	POSITION	PROPOGA-TION
Symphytum	P	1m	medium-heavy	sun-shade	root division
Tanacetum parth.	P	50cm	light-medium	sunny	seeds, division
Tanacetum vulg.	P	1.5m	medium-heavy	sun-shade	root division
Thymus	P	30cm	light, drained	sunny	cuttings division
Tussilago	P	30cm	medium-rich	sun-shade	root division
Valeriana	P	1.5m	medium-rich	semi-shade	root division
Verbascum	Bi	1.5m	medium-rich	sun	seeds
Vinca	P	50cm	medium, drained	semi-shade	cuttings

P = perennial   A = annual   Bi = biennial

CHAPTER NINE
Finding a Herbalist

TRADITIONAL HERBAL MEDICINE HAS ALWAYS BEEN HOME MEDICINE. That is to say the medicines themselves have been freely available to anybody choosing to harvest and prepare them. More recently, prepared herbal medicines have been available from good health food shops and many forwardthinking pharmacies. However, correct diagnosis of illness and the most appropriate choice of herbs does require skill. Many people prefer to consult a qualified medical herbalist. This means sound medical advice and the best advice on the best herbal prescription. But how can you find a herbalist?

Medical herbalists are not allowed to advertise their whereabouts, skills and wares as high-street chain stores and supermarkets do. This is because they are professions like doctors and solicitors. They can be found through easily accessible sources of information.

It is most important to ensure that, however you locate your herbalist, he or she is both adequately qualified and belongs to a professional body that regulates their profession. In the UK, properly qualified medical herbalists will have the letters MNIMH (Member of the National Institute of Medical Herbalists) or FNIMH (Fellow of the NIMH) after their name. To be a member, the herbalist must have taken a four-year medical course supervised by the Institute and passed all required exams, including a clinical exam where both doctors and qualified herbalists do the examining. Only after this qualification can their membership be considered. All members must follow a strict code of ethics and practice. The Institute maintains a complaints procedure. Any member of the public who is unhappy either with how a member of the Institute has behaved towards them or with any professional aspect of their treatment from a member, can lodge a complaint that will be investigated. This is an important safeguard for patients and is the same type of regulation and protection that exists with doctors.

How can you find out if a herbalist is a member or fellow of the NIMH? Ask. Don't be afraid of offending. Any member or fellow will be more than pleased to show you their card or even their certificate of membership. You could also write to the NIMH, who will send, free of charge, a copy of their register of members and fellows.

National Institute of Medical Herbalists
56 Longbrook Street
Exeter
Devon, EX4 6AH
United Kingdom

Members of the NIMH can be found around the world, but many countries have their own equivalent bodies. In Australia, for example, it is the National Herbalists Association of Australia.

Many people locate local herbalists through friends who are or have been patients. This is often useful as a recommendation carries confidence. But there are many other accessible routes to follow:

- Write to the National Institute asking for a register of members.
- The Yellow Pages phone directory usually lists herbalists under their own heading. Often members of the NIMH are grouped together, but if not they will have the letters MNIMH or FNIMH after their name.
- Look in local business directories. These are often distributed free to households or are in the public libraries. Look for a 'herbalists' heading as well as for local clinics or health centres of complementary or natural medicine where herbalists may be practising.
- Ask the receptionist at your local doctor's surgery. They often work closely with herbalists and may be able to recommend local practitioners.
- Ask at the public library or Citizens Advice Bureau. Both have lists of local services, including herbalists and other complementary health practitioners.
- Health food shops are an excellent source of information. Local practitioners may display their cards on notice boards in the shop or the staff may know who practises locally.

BIBLIOGRAPHY AND READING LIST

British Herbal Pharmacopoeia (1983), British Herbal Medicine Association, Bournemouth UK.

Fisher M.F.K. (1983), *A Cordial Water*, Chatto & Windus, London.

Grieve M. (1978), *A Modern Herbal*, Penguin, London.

Griggs B. (1981), *Green Pharmacy*, Robert Hale, London.

Griggs B. (1993), *The Green Witch*, Random House, London.

Hooper M. (1992), *Herbal and Medicinal Plants*, Rainbow, London.

Hutchens A.R. (1991), *Indian Herbology of North America*, Shambala, Boston & London.

Lasak E.V. and McCarthy T. (1987), *Australian Medicinal Plants*, Methuen Australia, North Ryde, Australia.

Mabey R. et al, (1988), *The Complete New Herbal*, Elm Tree Books, London.

Mills S. (1991), *Out of the Earth*, Viking Arkana, London.

Ody P. (1993), *The Herb Society's Complete Medicinal Herbal*, Dorling Kindersley, London.

Phillips R. and Foy N. (1990), *Herbs*, Pan, London.

Phillips R. (1977), *Wild Flowers of Britain*, Pan, London.

Polunin M. and Robbins C. J. (1992), *The Natural Pharmacy*, Dorling Kindersley, London.

Priest A.W. and Priest L.R., (1982), *Herbal Medication, A Clinical and Dispensary Handbook*, Fowler, London.

Robbins C.J. (1993), *Introductory Guide to Herbalism*, Thorsons, London.

Stockwell C. (1988), *Nature's Pharmacy; A History of Plants and Healing*, Century, London.

Trease G.E. and Evans W.C., (1983), *Pharmacognosy*, Twelfth edition, Baillière Tindall, Eastbourne UK.

Weiss R.F. (1988), *Herbal Medicine,* Arcanum, Beaconsfield UK.

Wren R.C. (1988), *Potter's New Cylopaedia of Botanical Drugs and Preparations*, Daniel, Saffron Walden, UK.

USEFUL ADDRESSES IN THE
UNITED KINGDOM

ORGANIZATIONS

National Institute of Medical Herbalists
56 Longbrook St
Exeter
Devon
EX4 6AH

School of Phytotherapy
Bucksteep Manor
Bodle Street Green
nr. Hailsham
Sussex
BN27 4RJ

University of Exeter
Centre for Complementary Health Studies
Streatham Court
Wrennes Drive
Exeter
Devon
EX4 4PU

British Herbal Medicine Association
PO Box 304
Bournemouth
Dorset
BH7 6JZ

The Herb Society
77 Great Peter Street
London
SW1P 2EZ

SUPPLIERS

Blackmores Limited
Unit 7
Poyle Technical Centre
Willow Road
Poyle
Colnbrook
Bucks
SL3 0DP

Cedar Health Limited
Pepper Road
Hazel Grove
Stockport
Cheshire
SK7 5BW

Culpepper Limited
Hadstock Road
Linton
Cambs
CB1 6NJ

Dorwest Herbs
Shipton Gorge
Bridport
Dorset
DT6 4LP

East West Herbs Ltd
Langston Priory Mews
Kingham
Oxfordshire
OX7 6UP

Bioforce (UK) Ltd
South Nelson Road
Cramlington
Northumberland
NE23 9HL

Frank Roberts (Herbal) Dispensaries Ltd
91 Newfoundland Road
Bristol
BS2 9LT

Gerard House Limited
457 Capability Green
Luton
LU1 3LU

GR Lane Health Products Ltd
Sisson Road
Gloucester
Gloucestershire
GL1 3QB

Healthcrafts Limited
c/o Ferrosan Health Care
Beaver House
York Close
Byfleet
Weybridge
Surrey

Phyto Products Ltd
3 Kingsmill Way
Hermitage Lane
Mansfield
Notts
NG18 5ER

Rutin Products Ltd
c/o Power Heath
10 Central Avenue
Airfield Estate
Pocklington
Yorks
YO4 2NR

Salus (UK) Ltd
15 Rivington Court
Hardwick Grange
Wollston
Warrington
Cheshire
WA1 4RT

INDEXES

To make it easier to use the information in the book, the index has been divided into five parts.

The GENERAL INDEX contains references to general information, for example on history of herbs, old herbals, common herbs, herbal medicine, etc. More detailed information is contained in the special subject indices. Some information will be found in both the GENERAL INDEX and the other indices, so looking in more than one index as appropriate may be useful.

The ACTIONS AND ACTIVE INGREDIENTS index contains references to the medicinal actions of herbs and the chemical ingredients that are responsible. The AILMENTS index contains references to specific discussions of important ailments and of both the herbalists approach to these ailments and some of the herbs that are used in treatment. Both herbal remedies that are used by professional herbalists and those suitable for household use are listed. The HOME–REMEDY KIT index lists all ailments and herbs discussed in the special chapter on using herbs safely and effectively at home.

The LATIN AND COMMON NAMES OF PLANTS index includes the MATERIA·MEDICA, a listing of all the important medicinal herbs that are discussed in detail.

These herbs are used regularly by professional herbalists and are both described and illustrated in their own chapter. Medicinal herbs are best referred to by their Latin names wherever possible. This is not to make life difficult. Common names can change in different parts of a country and more often between countries. Sometimes several different plants may even have the same common name, which can be confusing. The scientific or Latin names however are common to all languages and are the only plant names recognized throughout the world. The LATIN NAMES and COMMON NAMES included in this index allow easy reference to plant names, including all the text references to particular plants throughout the book.

GENERAL INDEX

A

abdomen: contents, 78
abortefacient, 125; herbs, 125
absinthe, 33, 182
acetic acid, 143
Achillea, 86, 88, 91, 92, 116, 146, 153
Achilles, 167
acne, 129–130; androgen hormones and, 129; herbal treatment, 129; herbs for, 130; period related, 129
Aconite, 162
Acontium, 98, 131, 142
acorns: pig and human food, 255
Acorus, 80, 81, 85, 123, 127
adaptogen, herb action, 105
adenoids, 117
adenovirus, 69
adrenal gland, 22; hormones released, 150

Ægopodium, 98
Aesculapius, 10
Aesculus, 86, 91, 92, 146, 152
Agrimonia, 83, 84, 120
agrimony, 49
Agropyron, 107
ague weed, 211
AIDS: herbs being researched, 206; research on herbs, 23
ajowan, 24
Alchemilla, 109, 110, 159
alcohol: and blood circulation, 92–93; and gastritis, 80; and pancreatitis, 85
alcoholic drinks and health, 33; herbs used, 34
alcoholic extracts, (see tinctures)
ales: herbs for flavouring, 225
alexander root, 25, 63
Alexander the Great, 174
alexanders, 37, 63

dock leaves, 57

doctors, 13–14; disputes with surgeons, 14

doctrine of signatures, 13

dog rose, wild, 39

dog's bite: ancient cure for, 177

dormouse: in *Alice in Wonderland*, 24

dose, 166; precision of, 140

doughnut: explains human body shape, 78

dropsy, 31, 56; causes of, 56; receipt for, 56; traditional remedy for, 204

drug: origin of term, 7

Druids: and mistletoe, 281

drying herbs, at home, 299–300

dulse, 37

Duncan I of Scotland, 183

duodenum, 80; ulcers of, 80

durian, 28

dye: yellow from hydrastis, 226

dyeing: methods, 49; with herbs, 49

dyer's broom, 19, 49

dyspepsia, 81; herbal treatment, 81; herbs for, 81; symptoms, 81

E

ear wax, 58

earache, 117

eardrum, 75; perforated, 76

earth worms, 58

Ebers papyrus, 10

Echinacea, 67, 69, 70, 71, 73, 79, 105, 111, 112, 117, 119, 123, 128, 130, 131, 155, 158

ectopic pregnancy, 111

eczema, 41, 126, 158; allergens, 126; and burdock, 37; atopic, 122, 126; contact, 122; discoid, 127; endogenous, 126; herbal treatment, 127–128; exogenous, 127; herbal treatment, 128; herbs for, 128; in ear canal, 75; of eyelids, 77; symptoms, 126; varicose, 127

Edinburgh Dispensary, 28

EFA, (see essential fatty acids)

Egyptian, 60

Egyptian pharaohs: cough remedies, 235; embalming fluids, 200

elder, 261; and superstition, 261; spirit, 32

elder flower, 38, 43, 44, 48, 59

elder leaf, insect repellent, 53

elder tree: berries, 53

elderberries, 49; ideal for children, 116

elecampane, 12, 60, 64, 117

Elettaria, 155

Elizabeth I, 14

Elutherococcus, 74, 79, 105, 112, 128, 130, 146, 160

emetics, 154; as expectorants, 154; herbs, 154; in poisonings, 154

emmenagogues, 159

emollients, 161; definition, 161; herbs, 161

emphysema, 73, 88; herbal treatment, 73; herbs for, 73; symptoms, 73

emulsifying ointment BP, 297

endocrine glands, 22

endometriosis, 109, 111; herbal treatment, 109

endoscope: diagnostic tool, 81

enuresis, (see bedwetting)

enzymes: digestive, 78

Ephedra, 72, 134, 152, 153

ephedrine, 148

Equisetum, 73, 74, 107, 108, 153

eringo, 58

Escherichia coli, 30

Eschscholzia, 103, 162

essential fatty acids, 143; and eczema, 127

essential nutrients, 19

essential oils, 23, 24; definition, 52; relaxing, 41; stimulating 41

eucalyptus, 64, 119; oil, 64

Euphrasia, 77

Euphrates, 9

Euphrosne: a Greek grace, 212

Eustachian tubes, 76, 117, 118

Evelyn, John: diarist on hops, 255; on balm, 239

H

Y

Z

ACTIONS AND ACTIVE INGREDIENTS

This index lists the actions of medicinal herbs that make them useful in healing and the main ingredients that are responsible for their therapeutic actions. The actions listed refer to herbs in the Materia Medica.

A

acetylcholine, 189, 276
acetylene derivatives, 269
actions of herbs, 148–162, 206, 261;
    digestive, 232
active ingredients of herbs, 143–148,
    192, 206, 245, 265
adaptogen, 207
adaptogenic, 245
adrenal cortex stimulant, 222
adrenogenic, 245
alkaloids, 148, 184, 186, 190, 193,
    194, 198, 208, 209, 218, 219, 226,
    231, 234, 235, 246, 247, 248, 249,
    266, 277, 283, 284; aconitine, 168;
    actinidine, 277, berberine, 186,
    198, 226; betonicine, 266;
    canadine, 226; capsaicin, 190;
    caulophylline, 193; cephaline, 195;

chatinine, 277; chelamine, 198;
chelerythrine, 283; chelidonine,
198; codeine, 246; emetamine, 195;
ephedrine, 168, 208; gelsedine,
218; gelsmedine, 218; gelsemine,
218; gentianine, 194, 218, 219;
gentioflavine, 194; harmaline, 247;
harman, 247; harmine, 247;
harmol, 247; hordenine, 284;
hydrastine, 226; isolobeline, 234;
lobelanidine, 234; lobeline, 234;
magnoflorine, 283; morphine, 212;
narcotine, 212; nicotine, 209;
nitidine, 283; norephedrine, 208;
oxycanthine, 186; palustrine, 209;
papaverine, 246; passiflorine, 247;
phytolaccine, 248; protoemetine,
195; sanguinarine, 246; sparteine,
168; stachydrine, 266; trigonelline,
266; valerianine, 277; valerine, 277

B

methylated flavonoids, 181
mild diuretic, 277
milletone, 250
minerals, 184, 207, 209, 276; calcium, 184; iron, 276; potassium, 276; silica, 184, 276
mood enhancer, 184
mucilage, 144, 171, 175, 181, 192, 196, 242, 251, 268, 272, 274, 275
mucilaginous polysaccharides, 196; isolichenin, 196; lichernin, 196
mustard oils, 180, 189
mydriatic, 183

N

narcotic, 183, 188, 246
nerve trophorestorative, 184
nervine, 184, 232, 256, 262
nervous tonic, 242, 266, 272
nutritive, 275

O

oestrogenic substances, 225, 260
oestrogenic, 222
oleanolic acid, 253
orexigenic, 178
organic acids, 251; benzoic, 251; fumaric acids, 251
oxalates, 258

P

painkiller, 168
paraciticide, 248
parturient, 242
pectin, 175
peripheral circulatory stimulant, 285
peripheral vasoconstrictor, 208
peripheral vasodilator, 205, 211
phagocytosis stimulant, 181
phenolic acids, 178, 182, 194, 202, 212, 219, 224, 241, 244, 260, 268, 236, 281; caffeic, 244; caffeic acid, 241, 260, 268; chlorogenic, 202,

268; rosmarinic, 244, 260, 268; vanillic acids, 241
phenolic compounds, 217; caffeic acid, 217; gaultherin, 217; salicylic acid, 217; vanillic acid, 217
phenolic glycosides, 259
phenols, 144, 285; gingerdiols, 285; gingerols, 285; shogoals, 285
phlobaphene, 252
picein, 259
piscidic acid, 250
plant acids, 143
polyacetylenes, 178, 206
polypeptides, 189, 257
polyphenolic acids, 210; caffeic, 210; gallic, 210
polyphenols, 239; caffeic acid, 239; rosmarinic acid, 239
polysaccharides, 206, 211, 270
pregnant uterus toner, 257
prostaglandin intermediary, 243
protein, 184
protoanemonin, 176
purgative, 174
pyridine alkaloids, 241; gentianine, 241
pyrollizidine alkaloids, 263, 268, 274; florosenine, 263; otosenine, 263; senescine, 263

R

ranunculin, 199
red pigment, 252
relaxant, 151, 233, 245, 272
resin, 174, 176, 177, 180, 186, 187, 188, 225, 226, 228, 234, 254, 256, 265, 280, 283; cannabinoids, 188
resins, commiphoric acids, 200; commiphorinic acid, 200
respiratory stimulant, 234
rhein, 192
rosmarinic acid, 240, 256
rotenoids, 250; rotenone, 250
rubifacient, 160–161, 180, 190, 210, 237, 256

AILMENTS AND THEIR REMEDIES

This index lists entries that describe or discuss ailments as well as relevant remedies.

HOME-REMEDY KIT

This index lists the herbs included in the home-remedy kit. Both main common names and Latin names are listed. More information can be found by looking up the herbs in the Materia Medica page 167–285.

A

C

D

E

F

LATIN AND COMMON NAMES
OF PLANTS

Latin names (family, genus and species) are in italics; common names in ordinary type; herbs included in the Materia Medica section are in bold italics.

B

balm, 239
Balotta nigra, 185
barberry, 186
batchelor's buttons, 269
bear's foot, 172
bearberry, 179
beargrape, 179
belladonna, 183
Berberis vulgaris, 186
Berberidaceae, 186, 193
bird pepper, 190
bitter wood, 249
bittersweet, 265
black cohosh, 199
black elder, 261
black haw, 278
black sampson, 206
black snake root, 199
black stinking horehound, 185
blackwort, 268
blé noir, 213
bloodroot, 252
bloody fingers, 204
blue cohosh, 193
blue gum, 210
blue rocket, 168
blue ginseng, 193
bogbean, 241
boneset, 211
Boraginaceae, 268
bottlebrush, 209
bread and cheese, 202
bridewort, 214
bruisewort, 268
bucco, 169
buchu, 169
buchweizen, 213
buckbean, 241
buckwheat, 213
bull's foot, 274
burdock, 178
Burseraceae, 200

C

cajaput, 237
Calendula officinalis, 187
cancer root, 248
Cannabinaceae, 188, 225
cannabis, 188
Cannabis sativa, 188
Cantheranthus rosaceae, 65
Caprifolicaeae, 261, 278
Capsella bursa-pastoris, 189
Capsicum minimum, 190
Carduus marianus, 145
Carduus marianus, 191
Carolina jasmine, 218
Caryophyllaceae, 267
casse lunette augentröst, 212
Cassia senna, 192
cassilata, 227
cat's foot, 221
catch grass, 216
Caulophyllum thalictroides, 193
cayenne, 190
Centaurium erythraea, 194
centaury, 194
Cephaelis ipecacuanha, 195
cetaria, 196
Cetaria icelandica, 196
Chamaelerium luteum, 197
chasteberry, 282
checkerberry, 217, 242
Chelidonium majus, 198
chickweed, 267
chilli, 190
Chinese ginseng, 245
Chondrus crispus, 37
Christ's ladder, 194
church steeples, 170
Cimicifuga racemosa, 199
cleavers, 216
clivers, 216
clot bur, 178
Cochlearia officinalis, 36
Cochleria armoracia, 180
cocklebur, 170
colic root, 205

S

T